MOVE A LITTLE, LOSE A LOT

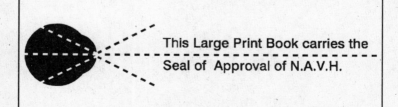

MOVE A LITTLE, LOSE A LOT

JAMES A. LEVINE, MD, PhD, AND SELENE YEAGER

THORNDIKE PRESS
A part of Gale, Cengage Learning

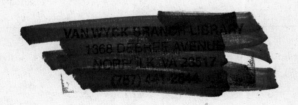
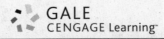
GALE
CENGAGE Learning™

Detroit • New York • San Francisco • New Haven, Conn • Waterville, Maine • London

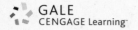
GALE
CENGAGE Learning™

Thorndike Press® Large Print Health, Home & Learning.

The text of this Large Print edition is unabridged.

Other aspects of the book may vary from the original edition.

Set in 16 pt. Plantin.

LIBRARY OF CONGRESS CATALOGING-IN-PUBLICATION DATA

Levine, James, 1963–
    Move a little, lose a lot / by James A. Levine and Selene
Yeager. — Large print ed.
        p. cm.
    ISBN-13: 978-1-4104-2817-2 (hardcover)
    ISBN-10: 1-4104-2817-6 (hardcover)
    1. Weight loss. 2. Reducing exercises. 3. Obesity —
Prevention. 4. Exercise — Health aspects. 5. Physical fitness.
6. Large type books. I. Yeager, Selene. II. Title.
    RM222.2.L4296 2010
    613.2'5—dc22
                                                    2010012586

Published in 2010 in arrangement with Crown Publishers, a division of Random House, Inc.

Printed in the United States of America
1 2 3 4 5 6 7 14 13 12 11 10

This book is dedicated to
Our children:
Ariella, Yael, and Juniper
And our long forgotten friend—the chair

ACKNOWLEDGMENTS

I wish to acknowledge the ever-present support of my workplace friends and colleagues and Heather Jackson and Eve Bridburg for bringing this book to life. I also wish to acknowledge the efforts of the team at Muve,* who is helping bring NEAT solutions to reality. I acknowledge the National Institutes of Health for funding the NEAT laboratory's research.

NEAT™ is a trademark and service mark of Mayo Foundation for Medical Education and Research.

The author's affiliation with Mayo Clinic does not constitute an endorsement by Mayo Clinic of the content of this book, or any views or opinions expressed in this book.

* Mayo Clinic owns equity in Muve, Inc. Mayo Clinic and James Levine, MD, PhD, may receive royalties from the sale of products developed and sold by Muve.

CONTENTS

9

■■■■

PART 1
THE SKINNY

■■■■

INTRODUCTION:
SENTENCED TO THE CHAIR

Have a seat. That used to be a polite invitation to take a load off your feet and rest awhile. But twenty years of researching the "science of sitting" has me thinking it's high time we changed that polite invitation to "Please, stand." Or "Come, let's walk."

Sitting was once a break in a busy day. Now it is the singular way most of us spend our time. Take a moment to reflect on a typical day. How did you get to work? Like 98 percent of Americans, you probably either drove or sat on a bus, train, or subway car. If you work in an office, the rest of your day was likely spent chairbound — at your desk, in endless meetings, or having lunch. What do you do after work? Sit down at the computer to pay some bills, shop online, catch up on e-mail? And after that? Maybe kick back and unwind with a few of your favorite shows?

Did you ever stop to think whether your

body was equipped to sit for thirteen, fourteen, fifteen, or maybe more hours a day? Did you ever consider what happens to your heart, muscles, and metabolism — that calorie-burning engine the fitness magazines are always advising us on how to "rev up" with green tea and exercise — when you sit virtually immobile for more than 80 percent of your waking hours?

Most of us haven't. We just accept it as the "way it is." But we never stop to realize that it's not the way it's always been or, more important, the way it was *meant* to be. We don't realize how stunningly recent this all-day sitting lifestyle is or the disastrous consequences it has had in just one generation's time.

Turn on some classic game shows like *Let's Make a Deal* from the late sixties and early seventies. Flip through some old photos from that time. Notice how practically "skinny" the average American looks compared to people today. Now flip on a football game or any show that provides a good wide-angle audience shot. Look at the general size difference from one generation to the next. The average American is 26 pounds heavier than they were back then. Two-thirds of us are now overweight. A third of us are obese. And we haven't just been getting fatter.

We've been ballooning to proportions once rarely witnessed except in scientific journals. Since the 1980s, the number of people who are more than 100 pounds overweight has skyrocketed to 4 million — one in every fifty adults — more people than live in the entire state of Colorado. By the end of the decade one in two children will be overweight. The past twenty-five years have brought us to a tipping point where for the first time in the history of mankind our life span has actually started to *decline* despite all recent medical innovation and progress. It's a case of chair today, gone tomorrow.

THE DIET AND EXERCISE LIE

If you're one of the majority of Americans who is overweight, you probably blame yourself for not exercising more or following the right diet. Why wouldn't you? Every magazine, infomercial, and weight-loss product sells special exercise plans and diets as the solution. Even the government spends millions of dollars promoting the diet and exercise message. It's not all bad, of course. But is it working?

Since 1972, when Dr. Atkins released his now-famous carb-eschewing opus, one big-name diet book after another has topped the charts. Atkins alone moved 45 million copies of his book during the past forty years. But are we any thinner? I have news for you: There's strong evidence that our calorie consumption has actually gone *down* or at least changed minimally during the past twenty years, as obesity rates have doubled. We also continue pouring stunning amounts of time and money into the exercise side of the equation, also to no avail. Since 1987, the number of health clubs in the United States alone has grown 146 percent to nearly 30,000 nationwide, while the ranks of members have swelled 58 percent to nearly 43,000,000. The weight-loss industry stands to rake in $58.7 billion this year, according to Marketdata Enterprises, a market research company in Tampa, Florida.

So each year we spend the equivalent of the gross national product of Bangladesh on slimming solutions, *and we're still getting fatter.* How much more money will we toss down this bottomless pit? How many more decades will we let this madness go on before we acknowledge that we're going about it all wrong?

Diet and exercise don't work because they are *unnatural.* Selectively eliminating entire food groups from your diet or eating only grapefruit or some special soup or shake is completely out of whack with the way we are

16

meant to live. Human beings are hardwired to eat to nourish ourselves, not to systematically deprive ourselves of sustenance. That's why you can never stay on a diet, and why you regain weight the moment you go off. We have evolved to hunt and gather, sow and reap, and to spend the day burning thousands of calories through constant motion, not to run like mad on a treadmill for 20 to 30 minutes, burning maybe 200 calories, and then sit nearly motionless for the other 15 1/2 hours of our day burning next to nil. That's why barely a quarter of the population regularly "exercises," and why half of all people who embark on an exercise plan abandon it within six weeks. We're simply not engineered to live like that.

I see patients time and time again who have reduced their food intake to pauper's portions and who go to the gym religiously, yet they still struggle with weight, hypertension, and high blood sugar. You know them, too. Maybe you are one. What does it all serve except to make you feel like a failure, and a hungry, irritable one at that?

Think about it. Could it really be that the *1 to 2 billion* overweight people spanning the globe have collectively grown so lazy and completely devoid of willpower in just one generation's time that they can't manage to follow one of the exercise or diet plans bombarding us all from every angle? No. Trying to tackle obesity through special diets and exercise is like trying to wag the dog. It plainly does not work.

As a doctor who has spent more than twenty years studying human movement, obesity, and metabolism, I can tell you that the way we are living and the way many of us are going about weight loss is absolutely, fundamentally wrong. Fifty years ago, there were no gyms; people rarely "exercised," and very few people struggled with being overweight. We managed our weight effortlessly because we *moved.* Now we struggle with it daily because we are desk sentenced.

NEAT: THE HUMAN ENERGY CRISIS

What happened between now and then? A profound energy crisis. That's what. Not fossil fuels like crude oil and gasoline (though as you'll see later, they *are* connected), but human energy — the very energy of life — the energy of my life's work: NEAT.

NEAT is short for an essential part of your calorie burning metabolism known as *nonexercise activity thermogenesis.* It sounds complicated, but it couldn't be more simple. NEAT is the calories (i.e., energy) you burn living your life. If you think of "exercise" as activity for the sake of developing and maintaining physical fitness, then NEAT is everything else. It's the calories you burn washing the car, walking to lunch, running errands, climbing the stairs, folding laundry, even tapping your toes and chewing gum. It is not going to the gym or taking an aerobics class. It is the energy we expend simply living. It's all the movements large and small we make throughout our day. Our current obesity and related health woes stem from the fact that modern life in the Internet-driven electronic age has increasingly leeched NEAT from our existence to the tune of up to 1,500 to 2,000 calories a day. And that loss is literally sucking the life out of us.

"I have no energy" is the number two complaint I hear from patients immediately after the number one complaint, "I need to lose weight!" It's ironic, isn't it? You spend all day sitting, which should leave you with energy to burn by the end of the day. Yet you feel completely and utterly spent and wanting nothing more than to collapse when you get home. My client Charlie, who lost 10 pounds of fat once he got off his seat and on his feet, said it best: "When I sit, sit, sit all day, the only thing I want to do is sit. I never had energy and didn't even know why. Now that I'm on my feet throughout the day, I'm more alert and energetic at work; and when I get home, I'm ready to go and play with my kids. My pants started to feel looser in just a couple of weeks. You can really feel the difference right away."

That is why I am writing *Move a Little, Lose a Lot,* to wake us all up out of our sedentary stupor and take us back to the healthy lifestyle we are born to live. We are so out of whack that it's as if we are fish living out of water. It's time to literally stand up for our health. I know you are probably thinking that there is little we can do to change our lifestyle because modern life and modern productivity demands hours upon hours of sitting. Well, I'm here to tell you that there is plenty we can and must do. And we can do it without sacrificing modern life. Indeed, we can do it without breaking a sweat or missing a work deadline. Fundamental lifestyle change is easier than you think. It just takes adopting a pattern of habitual, healthy behavior. A NEAT life filled with vibrant little movements infused into your day.

THE LURE OF THE NEAT LIFE

Up until a few years ago, I had a sedentary job as a scientist, stuck behind my computer all day. I figured I had the "good life," and my beer belly, fatigue, and frayed appearance were just part of the deal. Well, I thought it was the good life, until I met Pietro De'Sangiomiara, a barman at a hotel in Mexico City. I had just given a talk at an international conference and was ready to kick back at the bar. Pietro served up the best margarita you can imagine and we started chatting. He was about my age and looked (distressingly) wonderful — about 5 foot 9, lean, and suntanned — and he punctuated every sentence with a gleaming smile.

Pietro was married to Francine, who, according to his photo, was a Latin beauty. He explained the secret to keeping Francine happy was to keep him happy. He told me how he awakes at 9 a.m. or 10 a.m., when Francine brings him coffee in bed. Then, at 11 a.m. (his smiled implied how the hour between 10 a.m. and 11 a.m. was spent), they walk to her brother's or mother's house, where they have lunch, before walking to see friends or going home. Three afternoons a week, he plays soccer with friends from work. At four, he walks to collect the kids from school, and then he either plays with the kids or meets his brother. He has a light meal with his family before coming to work.

The only thing Pietro and I had in common was our love of soccer. I earned at least ten times more than he did, and he had at least ten times more fun. My NEAT burn at work was 400 calories a day; Pietro's was 1,500. Our jobs were radically different, of course. But we both worked ten hours a day. He just spent his ambling about, while I spent mine chained to a desk. In doing so, he easily expended 1,100 calories more than me. Comparing our leisure-time NEAT was nearly too depressing to bear. While Pietro was roaming about, making love, and playing soccer with friends, I was watching television until I switched screens and worked at the computer until I turned catatonic and went to bed. For my six hours of free time, I would expend about 30 NEAT calories, while he happily burned off thirty times that amount.

I wasn't quite ready to turn in my hard-earned MD, PhD career for a life of mixing mojitos in a cantina south of the border, appealing though it might sound, but it was clear that my good life had tremendous room for improvement, and it started with NEAT. Inspired by Pietro's constant movement, I completely reengineered my office in a way that got me off my duff and on my feet, yet still allowed me to get my work done. That was ten years and 30 pounds ago.

Since my own rebirth, I've helped thousands of people perform NEAT makeovers on their lives. Adopting a NEAT life is like rolling a boulder down a hill. The hardest part is getting it in motion; but once it gets going, it gains momentum until it's an irresistible force. I see it time and time again in my office. The world-weary man or woman walks in burdened with weight and saddled with the malaise of sedentary living. They often turn on me angrily when I offer a few simple NEAT solutions. Some even storm out.

Then they take that first step and the magic happens. NEAT begets NEAT. Take Gary, a fifty-nine-year-old construction supervisor. All he wanted to do was to be able to go down the slide at the park with his three-year-old grandson. But 60 excess pounds, diabetes, and joint pain made climbing playground equipment impossible. I advised him to find a place where he could insert ten minutes of NEAT activity in his day. He could start, I said, by simply getting up from his chair when his cell phone rang (which it inevitably did many times a day) and taking those calls standing and pacing. He did better than that. He told his boss to get rid of the shed he sat in all day while supervising construction sites. Instead, he chose to do the job on foot, walking among the workers instead of looking down from on high. Not only did he lose 45 pounds over the course of a year, but he also developed a stronger sense of camaraderie with his charges. With less weight came less joint pain and more energy. After years of miserably circling the drain in his life, he was joyfully climbing the ladder . . . and sliding down the slide.

Gary is just one example. I've seen the amazing power of NEAT living in my patients and in my lab at Mayo Clinic. As you'll soon read, I have documented proof that NEAT is what separates the lean from the obese. I have watched people with high NEAT consume tens of thousands of calories above and beyond what anyone should . . . and not gain a single ounce. I've seen clients lose 40, 50, even 60+ pounds and no longer need insulin because they adopted a NEAT-activated lifestyle.

MOTION IS THE NOTION

The NEAT Life is not another quick-fix diet or exercise plan that might dazzle in the short term, but will ultimately fail. No, I take the long view, focusing on the journey as opposed to the destination. *Move a Little, Lose a Lot* is about fundamentally changing your daily life in a way that will keep you fit and healthy year in and year out. It is based on real NEAT science that uncovers the way our human bodies are built and how they are meant to run. It shows you — in a step-by-step fashion — how to live the way those effortlessly lean people live and how to make it nearly effortless for yourself as well.

NEAT is more than my research or my passion of the moment. It is my life's work. My calling. I've been fascinated by energy and metabolism for as long as I can remember . . . even long before I knew what they were. As a chubby nine-year-old, I used to lie in the bath trying to calculate my calorie burn as my body expended energy heating the water. I spent hours trying to wrap my young mind around how I generated energy (and could maybe lose weight) with every flick of my wrist and wiggle of my fingers.

By age ten, I was beginning the experiments that have now culminated in this book, including one in which I placed fifteen pond snails in a self-made aquarium and tracked their movements every half hour during the night (I had to spend my days in school, after all), tracing their trails on wax paper each morning. One year and two hundred wax-paper trails later, I arrived at the same conclusion I would come to twenty-three years later — the energy of life,

NEAT, defines the function of an organism. NEAT isn't just something you choose. It is hardwired in your very cells. It is our biological imperative to move.

I followed this passion through college, where I studied clinical nutrition, into medical school, where I focused on internal medicine and endocrinology, and beyond medical school, where I earned a PhD devising instrumentation to measure the rate of human heat loss. I've devoted the past twenty years exclusively to NEAT and ultimately became the director of the NEAT Center at Mayo Clinic. My team includes 150 researchers, dietitians, and graduate students who study everything NEAT: in people young, old, lean, and obese; in populations; and within the brains of humans and animals. We study how microtechnology can be used to measure and change NEAT, and most important, we study how to change our world so that we can help people improve their lives. Our sole mission is to educate, motivate, and support people in adopting healthy, sustainable, weight-loss solutions, starting with NEAT.

I am proud to say that I have become a leading world authority on preventing and treating the global obesity epidemic. My work at Mayo Clinic has led to many publi-

In the spirit of NEAT living, I advise you to read this book standing up whenever possible. Pace around your house with it as you page through the contents. Place it on the kitchen counter and read on your feet while sipping your coffee. Take it to your son's soccer practice and leaf through it while you stroll. You'll not only burn more calories and rev your fat-burning metabolism, but also you'll process the information faster and more clearly, because, as you'll soon learn, even your brain works better on the move. There's no time like the present. Stand up for your health and start living the NEAT life today.

cations in journals such as *Science, Nature,* and the *New England Journal of Medicine,* among others. I lecture on obesity around the world and am a senior adviser to U.S. government agencies, the United Nations, China, and several countries throughout Africa. I've received more than fifty national and international science awards.

Cruise the halls of my lab at Mayo Clinic and you'll see a NEAT revolution alive and thriving as my colleagues hold walking meetings; perform NEAT Beats (activities designed to be done on the move); tally up their NEAT points; take advantage of NEAT monitoring devices, such as the Gruve; and implement the dozens of strategies you'll learn in this book. But it's not just happening here. I'm working with Wal-Mart, Best Buy, Nike, Steelcase, Apple, and other corporate giants and progressive Fortune 500 companies who are beginning to catch the wave. We performed a NEAT makeover on an entire corporation in Minneapolis. You'll find the employees' inspirational stories, struggles, and successes throughout the pages to come. But I can tell you this: Collectively, they lost 156 pounds, 143 pounds of body fat, nearly halved their triglycerides, lowered cholesterol 15 points, and enjoyed unprecedented productivity.

I'm not saying this to impress you, but to impress upon you that NEAT is not a gimmick. It is not a passing fad that will be forgotten before the next diet book rolls out. Rather, it is my life's work and passion forged into a detailed map to a healthier future. It's my legacy. I'm doing this for my kids, myself, and my patients. I'm doing this for you and your kids. We're all sick and tired of the unhealthy, sedentary lifestyle that's been thrust upon us. We all want to live a better life. I have the answer. It is NEAT. So simple, yet so powerful. It's time to live just as you were meant to live . . . on your feet.

1
OVERWEIGHT? DEPRESSED? YOU HAVE SITTING DISEASE
FREE YOURSELF FROM YOUR DESK SENTENCE AND RECLAIM YOUR HEALTH THROUGH NEAT LIVING

The biological need to walk is as much a part of your DNA as having an opposable thumb on each hand. Human beings literally evolved to walk. Go back 2 million years, when primitive people left the forest to explore the plains. As opposed to our knuckle-dragging ancestors who moved about on all fours like primates, these early explorers needed two long legs and a vertical spine to stride across the plains and see over long grasses to find food and avoid danger. We evolved over millions of years so we could walk about and see what the planet had to offer.

That walk lasted about 2 million years. As we spread across the earth on foot, we evolved from a simplistic race that holed up in caves and nourished ourselves with whatever food we could scrounge up to a complex species with magnificent inventions and flourishing crops. As a species constantly in motion, we harnessed our intelligence to capitalize on the earth's rich resources to sustain, shelter, and even entertain ourselves. We walked and explored. We walked and worked. We grew more sophisticated. We developed cultures and societies. For millions of years, we have literally been on a march toward ever-greater progress.

In the past fifty years — a blink of an eye in the history of all of humankind — we got so good at developing ingenious time- and labor-saving devices that we literally started running the world not from our feet as nature intended, but from our behinds. Our finely tuned human machine — the product of millions of years of perfection through evolution — is now short-circuiting as we've become completely glued to our chairs during the past ten to twenty years. Today, our bodies are breaking down from obesity, high blood pressure, diabetes, cancer, depression, and the cascade of health ills and everyday malaise that come from what scientists such as myself have named *sitting disease*.

TAKE A STAND AGAINST SEDENTARY LIVING

When I give lectures about sitting disease and electronic living, someone will inevitably accuse me of being a technology-hating Luddite. Make no mistake. I am a futurist, not a man who lives in the past. I marvel at every new piece of technology, and as a scientist and inventor I put modern electronic wizardry to good work every day in my lab. Indeed, as you'll later learn, I think the same technology that painted us into this sedentary corner will ultimately clear the path back to active living. But first we must realize what we've lost and how we lost it.

My research shows that the loss of NEAT from work and play can diminish our daily calorie burn by up to an astonishing 2,000 calories! But it's happened so gradually and subtly, we barely noticed it vanishing. To understand the magnitude of sitting disease and how to stand up to it, you have to look back at our history before we became chairbound.

At Work: From Cornfields to Cubicles

A pedometer study of an Old Order Amish community found the average man logged 18,000 steps per day — 9 miles — and the average woman logged 14,000 steps per day — 7 miles — while carrying out their daily litany of chores and other "to-dos." By contrast, the average deskbound American man and woman log a mere 5,000 to 6,000 steps — about one-third as many. Is it any wonder that as modern workers left the cornfields and took up the cubicles they collected countless unwanted pounds, while the Amish maintain the lowest rates of overweight and obesity of any community in North America?

This is not a call for us to go back to our agrarian roots or become a nation of step counters. NEAT is the buzz of human vibrancy, not simply "steps." But it is a call to reexamine the walled-in workplace.

It is no coincidence that "think outside the box" became such a popular turn of phrase since boxed-in cubicle-style workplaces became the norm. Remember the 1970s office? If you don't (or prefer not to admit you do), I'll take you back. Before cubicles — which were introduced in the mid-1960s — took over, shared offices were the norm, as were open floor plans with rows and columns of desks (imagine a bustling newsroom with phones ringing and typewriters clicking and you get the picture). Computers were just starting to creep into the mainstream, but most office tasks, from researching to filing to interoffice communication, were done by hand and foot.

Just twenty years ago, most every task of even white-collar work was an exercise in energy expenditure. Just getting to the job meant walking there, or at least to the bus, subway, or car-pool pickup. Spreadsheets and ledgers for accounts were literally sheets of paper you flipped through and penciled in. When you had research to do, you schlepped to the library and climbed the stacks with armfuls of books and microfiche. Billing problem? Off to search for Marge three floors down in the accounting department, who would inevitably be away from her desk when you needed her most, leading to multiple Marge-hunting sessions throughout the day. Important client to impress? Time to whip out a sharp X-Acto knife and start (literally) cutting and pasting (yes, people actually did that by hand before Microsoft Word and PowerPoint) together a snazzy poster-board presentation. If you wanted a colleague's impression on a work in progress, you had to get off your duff and step over to his workspace or rap on his office door. Files existed in large metal cabinets you wrestled open and hip-checked closed; cleaning them out was a daylong affair. When a report "absolutely, positively" had to be on your boss's desk the next day, you stood by the copier for what felt like an hour before you made a mad dash for the FedEx office to hurl it through the slot before last call at 6 p.m.

Even office socializing was more energetic. Standing around the water-cooler rehashing last night's game was a sport in and of itself, with wild gesticulations and collective scurrying back to work at the first sight of the boss. When it was time to round up the regular cast of characters for lunch, you literally did just that, made the rounds and swooped them out of their office spaces one by one as you meandered your way down to the cafeteria. Company bowling and softball leagues were popular ways to blow off steam when the day was done.

TO BUILD THE PERFECT CHAIR

Ever wonder why a simple-looking office chair can cost more than a basic treadmill? Because we're made to walk, not sit, and chair manufacturers have gone to great pains to keep us from protesting as our workplaces plant us there for longer periods of time. For $2,000 or more you can buy an "intensive-use" office chair that is specially designed with shock absorbers that support 500 pounds for five years, twenty-four hours a day, and that marries the contours of your body so you literally become one with the apparatus. You'll never feel like you need to move again . . . until you try to get up, that is.

How much has changed in a generation's time? Today, a mere 2 percent of us walk to work — less than half the number who commuted by foot just twenty years ago and ten times less than fifty years ago. Spreadsheets are banged out à la Excel. Surfing Google has replaced rummaging through library shelves. The most dynamic, dazzling dog-and-pony presentations are done with a few clicks of a mouse. Files are clickable icons on your desktop. Billing problems, colleague questions, and papers that need to be delivered are all sent in a matter of cyberseconds through e-mail and instant messaging. We riff about last night's game via e-mailed YouTube and ESPN links. Bowling leagues? Who has the time or the energy?

Even traditionally active jobs in the manufacturing industry (which is ever shrinking in the United States) have become increasingly sedentary as computers and robotics replace manual labor with machines.

Since we spend the majority of our waking hours at work, our loss of NEAT at the workplace has had the most profound effect on our energy expenditure. As you can see from the chart above, the NEAT expenditure we lose as we leave the fields and hole up in the office can add up to 1,500 to 2,000 calories each and every day — a full day's

Occupation Type	NEAT (kcal/day)
Chairbound	300
Seated work: no option of moving	700
Seated work: discretion & requirement to move	1,000
Standing work: e.g., homemaker, shop assistant	1,400
Strenuous work: e.g., agriculture	2,300

Data assuming BMR = 1,600 kcal/day

Black, *Eur J Clin Nutr* 50:72

worth of food for an adult woman or man.

That loss alone would be enough to toss a wrench into our movement-based metabolism. But we haven't only lost NEAT in our professional lives. It's been engineered out of other aspects of daily life to the point of near extinction. This creeping loss of activity happened so gradually that it's easy to imagine life always was as it is today. It doesn't take much digging to reveal the truth — or its consequences.

Home Improvement?

Did you wind your alarm clock today? Depending on your age, you might not even know what I'm talking about. From the time my father raised me to when I started raising kids of my own, the home has gone from a buzzing hub of domestic activity to a nest of NEAT-limiting devices. The alarm clock that wakes me is plugged in and pre-programmed, whereas the alarm clock my father used had to be hand wound every evening. My bathroom is next to my bed-room; my father had to use an outhouse (and later had the "luxury" of an indoor bathroom centrally located in the house). My coffee grinder is a push-button device, whereas my father ground his coffee using a hand-rotated mill. My shirt comes pressed from the cleaners, whereas my father's was hand ironed. Even my automatic machines have remote controls, so I don't even have to get up to push a button.

On any given Saturday or Sunday, it's pos-sible for me to have used more than forty "energy-saving" (read "NEAT-squelching") devices before I even think about leav-ing the house for the day: automatic alarm clock, cell phone, BlackBerry, home com-puter, espresso machine, microwave, clothes steamer, remote controls for the television, radio, and CD player, iPod, clothes washer, clothes dryer, electric toothbrush, automatic car starter, snowblower or lawn mower, electric dog fence, automatic dog/cat feeder, phone answering machine or service, house alarm system, air conditioner, push-button fireplace, pager, video gaming unit, hand-held video gaming unit, automatic icemaker, intercom, baby monitor, baby-bottle warmer, baby-wipes warmer, battery-operated screwdriver, food mixer, smoothie maker, bread machine, key finder, personal voice recorder, and the one I cannot live without, nose-hair clipper.

The irony is that these devices were devised to get the job at hand done more quickly and easily so we could have time and energy for other tasks, which in turn we could now do more quickly and easily to have more time for fun. Sounds good, until you realize that fun just isn't what it used to be either.

Go Fish . . . or at Least Watch It on TV

Having machines do all the work so we can play was a brilliant move. Unfortunately, the more energy we "saved" through technology and automation, the less we seemed to have for even the activities we once enjoyed. In just the past decade, our leisure activities have grown decidedly more leisurely. According to a poll of more than one thousand men and women, only 29 percent of American's current favorite pastimes involve any physical activity, down more than a third from ten years ago. Past favorites such as swimming, walking, and gardening have slipped from favor. Fishing and bowling are becoming quaint activities from bygone days. Even golf, a perennial American favorite, has been on a precipitous decline, with numbers dropping by the millions during the past decade.

It's not for a lack of free time. Believe it or not, surveys show that men and women today have almost five more free hours per week than we did in the sixties. Why does it feel like so much less? For one, we've become a nation of multitaskers, so every spare second is jam-packed. "Thanks" to technology, we can skim the news, chat with a friend on our cell phone, book our next business trip, and download new music without so much as standing up. While we do more, we move less. We also fill our free time with vampire activities that suck away time and energy without accomplishing much — like surfing the Web. Ever notice how you sit down to Google something, only to look up and see an hour has evaporated?

For many of us, playtime has come to mean "screen time." Surveys show that television watching and Internet surfing (often done simultaneously) are overwhelmingly our favorite form of entertainment. The average American flicks on the tube and watches as

41

much as *five-plus* hours of television each day, according to a study from Ball State University, where researchers sat in people's homes and logged their screen time.

I am not one of those fanatical doctors who condemn television as evil. It does serve a very important function in providing information and allowing us to shut down our brains after a busy day (a good sitcom does it for me every time). But that's the point. We abuse TV's great power. Television viewing does more than slow NEAT; it literally shifts it in reverse. Studies show brain waves fall into a slumbering state when you're staring at the screen. Just watch how motionless a group of otherwise rowdy children become when under the spell of their favorite show and you'll see what I mean. With a full 70 percent of our leisure fun now completely NEAT free, it's little wonder we feel so relentlessly tired and stressed. Our leisure-time activities no longer recharge our energies, but sink them into a state of depletion.

When we do get active during our leisure time, we now call it "working out." Sound like fun? Forget fun for a minute. Does it even make sense? Of course, athletes and gym-a-holics can burn a couple thousand calories a day in their exercise-centric existences; these, however, are hardly "average people," and as you'll soon see "exercise" does not necessarily make you "active." Somewhere along the line, everyday people abandoned their active NEAT play — the types of enjoyable pursuits such as boccie and bowling that easily expend a few hundred NEAT calories — for "working out" at the gym. The catch is that unlike fishing, gardening, golf, knitting, and bridge playing, which provide pleasant, social escapes, most people consider gym exercise an obligation from which they would rather escape . . . most likely to the TV.

Stuck in Overdrive

In the 1950s, few Americans owned cars. Over the past few decades, car ownership has grown from zero to the present state where the vast majority of families own at least one, and often two or more, cars. In fact, three-car garages are becoming a mainstay of the American suburban home. Car manufacturers sell us on the NEAT of cars — the lure of buzzing down the open road in your Chevy or 4Runner, the speed, the adventure, the wind in our hair, left arm dancing out the window on top of the rushing breeze blowing by. But the reality is we are locked in our cars creeping along at a near standstill (often angrily), snarled in traffic, belching out exhaust and becoming further isolated, exhausted, and sedentary.

The massive upswing in obesity rates during the past forty years matches the number of miles per day the average person travels by car in the United States. That is, we now drive an average of 30 miles a day and weigh roughly 30 pounds more than we did in 1960. That's not terribly surprising when you figure that walking to work burns about 100 to 150 calories per half hour versus the 32 burned during a typical thirty-minute commute.

There are now 600 million cars on the road worldwide, with more joining the global traffic jam every day. And a car is now much more than a vehicle to carry us from point A to point B. Our Fords and Subarus serve as offices, living rooms (complete with DVD), and dining rooms (where the majority of our take-out meals are consumed). The car has become a crucial symbol of social status, and now sadly also a definer of the status of our personal well-being and that of our global health and environment.

It is projected that there will be 1 billion cars in use by 2020 — eerily parallel to the number of obese people in the world. The double-digit growth of the car market is especially pronounced in China. Crossing the thoroughfares in Beijing is now a matter of car avoidance, whereas ten years ago it was a case of avoiding being hit by a wave of bicycles. Interestingly, in China, one in six bicycles are now sold with an electric engine. Guess what? About one in five people in China are now overweight. Among those between thirty-five and fifty-nine years of age, that number rises dramatically, to 50 percent. As traffic rises, so do highway jams, and the number of hours we are spent stuck in our bucket seats.

Don't Get Up!

That's the NEAT-killing message permeating society today. For pennies a day, you can have everything from the latest Oscar-winning DVD movie release to your groceries and dry cleaning delivered directly to your door. Weekend football bonanzas can be enjoyed in a chair complete with cooler and snack tray, so you don't have to rise from the cushion to pop another beer. Web-based services will deliver lunch straight to your cubicle. At every turn, a new product or service steals a little bit more movement from your life. I was sitting in a coffee shop the other day and saw a poster advertising a new soft drink with a woman on a hammock declaring: "Life's better on the porch."

Is it? You might argue that it is wonderful you can earn money for the mortgage by merely flicking your wrists and fingertips all day, that a simple tilt of your ankle can transport you tens of thousands of miles each year, and that all you need do to put food on your table is roll down your car window and say, "Number 3 with a Coke, please." And it would truly be wonderful if our bodies were meant to operate this way. The trouble is, they're not. By meeting all of our needs on invisible networks, in gas-driven motor vehicles, and with high-convenience, zero-prep food, our bodies do not get the opportunity to realize their natural tendency to move. The consequences of denying our DNA go beyond diminished calorie burn, though the effect on our metabolism is unquestionably catastrophic. I see it every day in my office.

MORTGAGING YOUR METABOLISM

Jean was a classic client. She walked into the office where I was working as an intern; she was 40 pounds overweight with an equally heavy chip on her shoulder. She was seemingly angry with the world for making her overweight, and she wanted answers.

"I have four kids. My husband travels. When am I supposed to exercise and how can we *not* eat fast food?!" she said defensively before I so much as uttered a word. As I started explaining about NEAT, it sent her straight over the edge she was perched upon so precariously. "I have FORTY pounds to lose! I have tried every diet there is. I am not going to waste my time on all this small stuff!"

But like the soft, scrambled blur you see when standing too close to a Monet, Jean couldn't absorb the impact of these small actions because she couldn't see the big picture. It's completely understandable. Taken piece by piece, pulling and pushing a filing cabinet open and closed, crocheting a cap, chatting around the watercooler, and walking to the mailbox seem almost infinitesimal in the grand scheme of energy metabolism. But they are far more important than most imagined. Over time, they add up to massive amounts of calories burned.

To help Jean (and other clients) see the magnitude of NEAT, I use a simple financial analysis to which we can all relate: the mortgage. Let's say my paycheck is $3,000 a month. About 60 percent of that gets sucked up by basic home-ownership expenses, such as the mortgage, heat, and lights. About 10 percent, around $300 a month, goes to food. The rest, $900, is my disposable income, to spend how I choose. What I don't spend goes straight into savings. That's a good thing with money. It's not so great when it's calories.

How you expend calories is similar to how you spend money. The largest chunk (about 60 percent) goes to your basal metabolic rate (BMR). Those are the calories your body uses even when you are perfectly still to keep your heart pumping, your brain thinking, and all your organs doing their jobs. Similar to a mortgage, the bigger your "house" (i.e., body), the larger your BMR. Another, much-smaller number of calories are burned in what is called the thermic effect of food (TEF), a fancy way of saying the calories you burn digesting what you eat. TEF accounts for about 10 percent of your metabolism and doesn't vary very much. The final way you expend calories is movement — both purposeful exercise and NEAT, all those little movements we've been talking about. Physical movement accounts for about a third of the calories you burn each and every day. If you're like three-quarters of the population and do little purposeful exercise, *all* your additional calorie burn depends upon NEAT. For graphic purposes, I've illustrated the various forms of calorie-burning metabolism in the chart below.

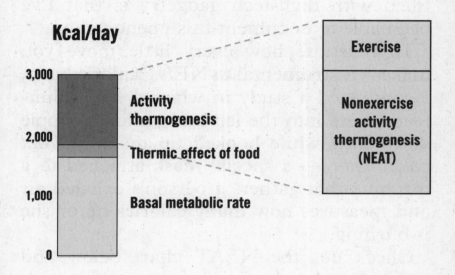

Kcal/day

3,000

Activity thermogenesis

2,000

Thermic effect of food

1,000

Basal metabolic rate

0

Exercise

Nonexercise activity thermogenesis (NEAT)

What happens if you remove purposeful exercise from the chart above? You lose what? One hundred calories? Not much in the big picture of human metabolism, especially if you exercise just three or four days a week. This distresses my patients who desperately carve out that twenty or thirty minutes to exercise. But unless you're exercising at a very high level or for a longer time, the calorie burn usually comes in at 100 to 200 — an amount easily erased by a few sips of frappuccino or a handful of M&M's.

Now remove NEAT from that chart. What's left? I'll tell you what's left: sitting disease and the obesity, diabetes, heart disease, and general malaise that accompany it. The marvelous thing about having a lab filled with high-tech gadgetry is that I've been able to document this phenomenon.

To illustrate how every little move you make is instrumental to NEAT calorie burn, I conducted a study in which I had volunteers come into the lab and perform simple daily tasks while hooked up to an *indirect calorimeter* — a special mask attached to a machine that gathers a person's exhaled air and measures how many calories he or she is burning.

Check out the NEAT chart below and watch what happens as the average volunteer goes from sitting still as a stone to standing to briskly walking. The mere act of standing on your feet burns three times as many calories as sitting in your seat. Any little movement on top of that (even something as minute as chewing gum!) creates even greater metabolic spikes. When you walk, your metabolism literally blasts off. Examining the chart, it's easy to see how the loss of constant daily activity has decreased our natural calorie-burning metabolism by more than 50 percent.

Here's another wonderful snapshot of NEAT in action, which came to me cour-

My client Maria does a superb job of blocking off three days during the week when she goes to the gym. She leaves work at 12:15 sharp and drives to the gym to arrive at 12:25. She changes quickly and is perched on the exercise bike by 12:30, where she pedals like mad until 1:00. Through the sweat and pain, she looks down at the display on the bike to observe just what she sees every time — she has expended 120 calories. She curses at the machine as she sprints to the shower at 1:01. At 1:10, she jumps into her car to race back to work, miraculously completing a one-handed, rearview mirror hair and makeup replenishment. She pants into work and retires back to her desk for the day at 1:20. For her dedication, she burns 360 calories a week — what averages out to 70 calories a day — an amount she could easily triple by boosting her NEAT.

tesy of Marc Hamilton, PhD, at the College of Veterinary Medicine, University of Missouri. This electromagnetic imaging chart shows muscular activity throughout the body as a volunteer sits, stands, and then takes

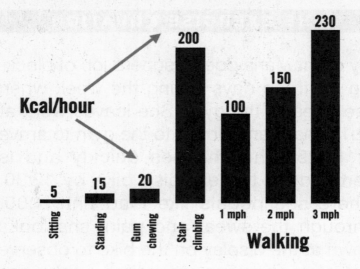

Kcal/hour

| 5 | 15 | 20 | 200 | 100 | 150 | 230 |

Sitting — Standing — Gum chewing — Stair climbing — 1 mph — 2 mph — 3 mph

Walking

a few steps across the room. Notice how muscular activity spikes during four simple steps (hardly enough to be considered "exercise"). Notice how much energy it takes just to stand up from a chair? Now look at how little muscle activity you generate while you sit. These are the scientific discoveries that have human metabolism researchers concerned that even "active" people in today's society are falling prey to sitting disease.

How can you be active and still have sitting disease? Let's say you got up this morning and jogged two to three miles for twenty to thirty minutes, then drove to work, where you sat for the next nine or ten hours before coming home and cementing yourself into the sofa for the evening. Then ask yourself:

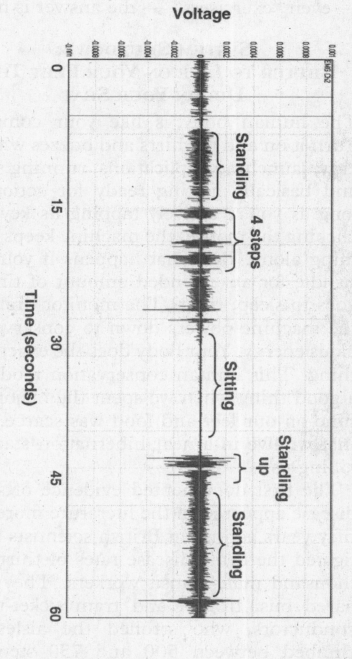

Provided by: Dr. Marc T. Hamilton, University of Missouri.

53

"Am I really active?" For far too many of us — even "exercisers" — the answer is no.

SYSTEM SHUTDOWN: BETTER TO LIVE ON YOUR FEET THAN DIE ON YOUR SEAT

The human body is like your computer. Turn it on and it whirrs and buzzes with energy, launching applications, running scans, and basically getting ready for action. So long as you're actively tapping its keys and clicking the mouse, the machine keeps humming along. But what happens if you let it sit idle for an extended amount of time? It goes to sleep, right? The monitor dims and the machine powers down to conserve precious energy. Your body does the exact same thing. This human conservation mode was a good thing when we spent the majority of time on our feet and food was scarce. Now that we live in a near hibernation state, it's killing us.

The first documented evidence of sitting disease appeared in the literature more than fifty years ago when British scientists investigated the heart disease rates of thirty-one thousand male transit workers. They compared bus, trolley, and tram ticket-taking conductors, who strolled the aisles and climbed between 500 and 750 steps per day, and the vehicle drivers, who sat behind the wheel for more than 90 percent of their shift. The outcome surprised even the scientists. The sitting drivers suffered three times the rate of coronary occlusion (the coronary artery blockage that can lead to heart attack) and more than twice the rate of death after a cardiovascular event such as a heart attack than the conductors who spent their working hours on their feet. Various reviews of activity on the job among other workers, such as post office employees and longshoreman, mirrored these findings. The conclusion: Physically active work protected against heart disease.

Now, more than fifty years later, the scientific community is finally starting to understand *why* sitting is so bad for you. There's a whole new realm of scientific study that is focusing not on activity, but rather inactivity, the science of prolonged sitting, and its metabolic consequences. The results have been stunning, even to me, who has studied NEAT for more than twenty years. As you'll soon learn, you actually have "NEAT cells" in your body that don't really respond to vigorous exercises such as running and step aerobics, but instead respond *only* to the gentle muscle contractions of NEAT — the simple movements of living. When those cells go neglected, even for short periods of time, the many incarnations of sitting disease can follow. Conversely, when you "shake your mouse" and get up out of your seat, those cells spring into action and put you on the road to optimum health . . . and happiness. Study after study proves that NEAT is the key to a longer, healthier, happier life.

NEAT Helps Your Heart

When I met Jerry, he was an office worker who looked every one of his forty-eight years. He hated how lethargic he always felt, hated the constant sitting, and had become increasingly worried about his health as his

THE GAME OF LIFE

Just how inactive has electronic living rendered us? Consider that a fourteen-year-old boy in England developed deep vein thrombosis (DVT), a potentially life-threatening condition caused by blood clotting in the legs that is usually seen in the elderly and infirm, after a ten-hour marathon session of video games one afternoon. Ironically, many video games today are designed with "endless lives" so you never have to stop and start over when your character dies.

weight crept ever closer to the 200-pound mark and his cholesterol level climbed to 260. Then he started following the NEAT plan (which you'll find later in this book). In six months, he lost 20 pounds of fat, gained 5 pounds of muscle, nearly halved his body fat, from 25 percent to 13 percent, and lowered his cholesterol more than 60 points, so it is now in a heart-healthy range. When I saw him six months after he started the plan, he looked like a new man, easily twenty years younger. He felt younger, too . . . a lot younger.

"I feel like I'm eighteen," said Jerry. "I wake up in the morning with endless energy. I never thought I would see 175 pounds again. The best part is you really don't have to do a lot. I don't eat perfectly. But by getting up and moving throughout the day, I have plenty of energy to stay active when I get home. I feel great."

As Jerry's example shows, NEAT is one of the best things you can do for your health, especially your heart. It starts at the cellular level. Your capillaries — which, as you know, are tiny blood vessels that deliver oxygen and nutrient-rich blood into tissues throughout your body — are lined with special cells called endothelial cells that assist the flow of blood. These cells contain an enzyme called lipoprotein lipase (LPL). Its job is to break down fat molecules (i.e., triglycerides) in the blood. As you might imagine, that's a very important job, since, unchecked, these blood fats are one of the leading triggers of heart disease. When you sit for a few hours, these enzymes start to switch off. Sit for the entire day and their activity levels plummet by 50 percent. Eat a high-fat meal after a day of sitting and you can watch your blood fats skyrocket 180 percent.

The mere act of getting up out of your chair is all it takes to break out of hibernation mode and switch these enzymes on again. We're not talking about getting up to go for a jog; we're just talking about getting up. In fact, research suggests that standing and light NEAT activity charge these enzymes and raise metabolism in a way vigorous exercise cannot. Vigorous activity only increases LPL activity in what are known as your "white" muscle fibers — those special fast-twitch muscles you use during hard exercise. It does little for the vast majority of your "red" slow-twitch muscles that are responsible for the NEAT activity in life — the muscles you use to simply stand, hold your body upright, and walk around. That is why walking and NEAT activity *every single day* is so essential, whether you're a couch potato, a weekend warrior, or a regular exerciser.

By getting up out of your chair throughout the day, you use a tremendous amount of energy over time. You engage postural muscles that "switch on" genes that are essential for good health. When you sit all day, your health goes into decline. A landmark study of more than seventy-three thousand women reported that risk of dying from heart disease was nearly three times higher among people who sit the most compared to those who sit the least. All-day sitting raised heart disease risk in both old and young, exercisers and couch potatoes. Another study concluded that prolonged sitting doubles your risk for metabolic syndrome — a constellation of risk factors for heart disease and diabetes, including high blood pressure, high cholesterol, high blood sugar, overweight (especially in the abdominal area), and high triglycerides. Among women, the risk for metabolic syndrome increases 26 percent for every additional hour they spend watching TV. The good news: Every thirty minutes spent in NEAT activity provides a similar degree of protection.

Need more proof? In a fascinating study done at Harvard, researchers followed more than fifteen hundred women for nearly thirty years to investigate how physical activity helped prevent heart disease. Along the way, they tracked their energy expenditure from how many flights of stairs they climbed, how much they walked, what sports they played, and what type of exercise they performed in their spare time. In the end, the activity that provided the most profound protection against heart disease was walking. Those who walked the equivalent of just ten blocks a day lowered their risk by 33 percent. Similar studies by the same research team found that walking just one hour a week was enough to reduce heart disease risk 20 percent.

These are just more clear examples of why exercise as we've come to know it isn't the answer. It's not bad for you. Indeed, it's quite healthy. But it doesn't replace NEAT. It doesn't replace the hundreds of thousands of muscle contractions your body needs throughout the day every day to burn calories and keep your body running and operating at its healthy best.

NEAT Shrinks Your Belly

Matt, a tall, soft-spoken forty-three-year-old businessman, held out the waistband of his pants proudly, exposing a 4-inch gap between his flattened abdomen and where his pants used to sit. "I'm going to need a tailor," he said with a smile. Matt started the NEAT plan because he wanted more energy to keep up with his two young children. He finished it 16 pounds and 7 percent body fat lighter, most off his midsection.

NEAT activity seems to tap into your belly fat stores first, which not only helps you look better on the beach, but it also extends your life. In a large international study of nearly 170,000 men and women in sixty-three countries, researchers have found that your belt size is the best indicator of your overall health and your risk for heart disease, diabetes, and death. Mirroring those findings, the Nurses' Health Study of more than 44,000 women also reported in the same journal (*Circulation*, the journal of the American Heart Association) that the bigger your waistline, the higher your risk of dying. Women whose waistlines were 35 inches or more were twice as likely to die of heart disease or cancer than those whose waistlines were less than 28 inches, even when their body mass index (BMI) fell within a normal, "healthy" range.

A waist circumference, which is the measurement straight around your navel, of greater than 32 inches in women and 37 inches for men raises the risk for heart attack, stroke, and diabetes. Women with a waist measurement of more than 35 inches and men whose belt size exceeds 40 inches are considered high risk for these and other diseases.

How can a little potbelly be so dangerous? Because unlike fat that pads your hips and legs, this fat sits around your internal organs and is metabolically active. It actually acts like a separate — and rather sinister — organ, pumping out its own hormones and interfering with the function of your liver. The result of all this mayhem is high triglycerides, unhealthy cholesterol levels, and high blood sugar. As if that weren't bad enough, this fat also interferes with appetite-regulating hormones, so you're inclined to eat more and store more fat, creating a vicious cycle.

Breaking free from this perilous downward spiral is as simple as standing up and taking a leisurely walk around the block. Belly fat cells respond quickly to even small amounts of movement, so even the smallest amounts of NEAT activity will help you shrink your waistline fast. A recent six-month study of 464 women reported that women doing the equivalent of just ten minutes of walking a day shrunk nearly 2 inches off their waistlines, even when they didn't lose weight. Within just two or three weeks of starting the NEAT plan, you will likely notice your clothes fit better, especially around the waist. By the end, you'll likely be like Matt, shopping for new belts . . . or a tailor.

Beat Fatigue with NEAT

"But Dr. Levine, I'm already so tired, I don't know how I could possibly be more active each day!" That is the lament I hear from many a client. My answer is always the same: "That's exactly why you *need* to be active more each day!" Unlike vigorous exercise that can leave you feeling wiped out and in need of a rest, NEAT activity has the opposite effect. It leaves you abuzz with energy. Science confirms it.

In a recent study on how exercise can be used to treat fatigue, University of Georgia researchers assigned thirty-six inactive men and women who complained of persistent fatigue to one of three groups. The first group did a moderate-intensity exercise, such as brisk walking uphill, for twenty minutes three times a week; the second group performed an easy activity, such as a leisurely walk, for the same time period; and the third group had no activity. After six weeks, both exercising groups enjoyed a 20 percent boost in energy while the sedentary folks stayed the same. But here's the really interesting part. The low-intensity group reported a 65 percent drop in feelings of fatigue, while the more intense exercisers had just a 49 percent drop.

This type of low-level NEAT activity is energizing because it stimulates the central nervous system, concluded the researchers, which is *exactly* what the NEAT buzz is all about! You feel better. You think more clearly (more on that in a bit). You have more vibrancy and zest. That's the NEAT life.

NEAT Builds Strong Muscles and Ache-Free Joints

It's not just your heart that suffers the consequences of too much sitting. All your organs, indeed, every cell in your body — needs NEAT. Like many people, however, your heart and internal organs may be a little too "out of sight, out of mind" to motivate you to move more. They don't protest loudly enough (until something's really wrong). But how about your back? Or your neck, hips, and knees? I bet they let you know how they feel without enough NEAT. Whoever coined the term *sitting pretty* clearly didn't sit for too long.

Sitting is a major cause of orthopedic pain. When you sit for extended periods of time, the muscles that hold you upright loosen, so they can't support your back as well. Meanwhile, your hips get tight and start pulling on your spine as you try to stand and walk. The end result is a hunched-over, head-forward posture that not only begins to resemble the Cro-Magnon man we walked away from a few million years ago, but also leaves you susceptible to debilitating back pain and injury. Likewise, your legs grow stiff and weak, leaving your knees vulnerable to the same aches and pains.

NEAT helps you move with greater ease even if you already have painful joints from arthritis. The Arthritis Foundation acknowledges that experts used to advise against activity, lest it further damage the joints. But now we know that daily activity is an essential tool in reducing joint pain, building strong muscles to support the joints, and improving range of motion and endurance.

STAND UP FOR YOUR HEALTH

Adam Campbell, the sports and nutrition editor at *Men's Health*, isn't one to take things sitting down. So when he developed chronic muscle imbalances in his shoulders and hips and nagging pain in his neck and back from hunching over a keyboard twelve hours a day, he dumped his chair and had his company outfit his office with an "SUD" — a stand-up desk.

At first, he was worried he wouldn't be able to work as well standing as sitting, a fear that dissolved as quickly as the incessant aches in his neck and back. "Standing up seems to improve my concentration. I think it's partially because it gives me a greater sense of urgency. When you're standing, you don't really relax, which helps you to avoid losing focus. And I have to say, my back, neck, and hips already feel better. So while you might think I'd get tired of standing, it's actually just the opposite. I like it a lot," said Campbell.

The pain relief isn't some placebo effect of Campbell's imagination. In a recent *USA Today* article on beating back pain, Stover Snook, who has lectured on ergonomics at the Harvard School of Public Health for thirty years, recommends eating breakfast standing up and, if possible, to work as Thomas Jefferson and Winston Churchill did — using a stand-up desk.

As a bonus, you just might shed some stubborn pounds. After writing about his SUD experience, Campbell received a wave of replies from readers who opted to work on their feet as well. One lost 35 pounds in a year by doing nothing more than trading his seat for his feet. And the trend seems to be spreading. Details (a major office furniture manufacturer) reports that "sit-to-stand" desks, desks you can raise high enough to work on while standing up, are their fastest-growing product category.

NEAT Makes You Smarter and Happier

Just as NEAT is about more than having flat abs, trim thighs, or even a healthy heart, the consequences of sitting disease extend far beyond your belt size or the numbers on the bathroom scale. Having NEAT stripped from your life literally stagnates your mind and robs your brain of the stimulus it needs to do its most basic job — problem solve.

Anyone who works a traditional desk job has likely witnessed this hundreds of times. You sit at your desk for hours desperately struggling to decipher a vexing dilemma or craft a brilliant memo, to no avail. Then the moment you toss your hands up in defeat, leave your desk, and march to the café for more coffee, the answers begin to flow seemingly effortlessly into your brain. How many people say their best ideas come to them in the shower? This is NEAT in its purest form. Human beings are meant to create on the move. We are hardwired to do our best exploring, inventing, and developing through the motion and energy expenditure of our human machine.

Albert Einstein, arguably the greatest thinker this world has known, was the perfect example of a mind in motion. His most brilliant, far-reaching construct — the very theory of relativity — did not come to him while parked on a chair. When asked how he came up with the now famous $E = mc^2$, he simply replied, "I thought of that while riding my bike," as though it couldn't have occurred to him any other place.

Aristotle knew it. His Peripatetic school was so called because he believed that philosophical quandaries were best sorted out *peripateo* — walking about the shaded pathways of the campus. He didn't sit stagnant with his students; they absorbed his lessons as they strolled. Even when he lectured in a classroom setting, he was known to pace — precisely what humans did to jar their minds into action before cubicles confined them to spaces barely suitable for standing, let alone ambling. Creative human thought is inextricably linked to movement . . . and vice versa.

Though we don't understand all the body-mind science behind NEAT and creative thought, we do know this: NEAT triggers brain growth. That's right. While NEAT activity shrinks your belly, it bulks up your brain. Beginning as early as your twenties, your brain begins to shrink and continues to diminish as you get older. Until recently, it's been considered an inevitable part of cognitive decline. Now scientists at the University of Illinois have found that as little as three hours of brisk walking a week is enough to boost blood flow to the brain and trigger biochemical changes that increase the production of new brain neurons. In one study, sedentary people who started walking increased their brain volumes to levels similar to people three years younger after just six months. This growth is especially pronounced in the frontal lobe and hippocampus, parts of the brain that govern memory, multitasking, and decision making.

NEAT makes you smarter, sharper, and more creative; yet today our minds are forced to work in a motionless environment. Obviously, we *can* work that way. We've been forced to do so. But if current mental health trends are any indication, we're none too happy about it.

Do you take antidepressants? If you don't, you surely know someone (at least one someone) who does. In 2000, the United Nations warned of an "alarming" rise in depression at work. Stress, anxiety, malaise, and depression on the job affect one in ten workers worldwide and cost employers in Europe and the United States $120 billion a year, according to the International Labour Organization.

Why so much sadness and despair in nations, such as the United States and Britain, where people have enjoyed relative prosperity? Because we simply can't cope with the pressures of a technology-driven economy that forces us to be absolutely sedentary yet enormously productive day in and day out. Our life force is stifled, while demands on our creativity and productivity are at an all-time high. Worse, we're imposing the same NEAT-crippling lifestyle on our children. Childhood obesity is expected to reach 50 percent in a decade. Given the toll sedentary living exacts on our mental health, it is no surprise that during the past thirty-five years, the rise of attention-deficit/hyperactivity disorder (ADHD) has surged among our children at unprecedented rates. Why? Because children, even more than adults, crave NEAT, as they fidget, dash about, and naturally move spontaneously throughout the day. Now that they're bused and driven to school and recess and phys ed have been diminished, their NEAT has been reduced. What is increasing are the prescriptions for Ritalin. In fact, one of my clients recently told me that since she started living NEAT with her family, her nine-year-old son, who has ADHD, has improved tremendously. "He has so much more focus now; it's been wonderful," she said. The best part: It's all from simply walking and playing more.

To be clear, I am not opposed to psychotropic medicines. For those who need them, they can be a lifeline out of despair. But a tall body of evidence shows that daily activity alleviates depression more quickly, just as effectively, and provides more long-term relief than drugs. In one striking study by Duke psychiatry professor James Blumenthal, PhD, researchers found that thirty minutes of activity just three days a week worked as well as antidepressants in a group of 156 adults. More important, those who regularly moved their bodies were much less likely to have their symptoms return six months later than those who relied on medication.

Unlike modern mood meds that work on one level — usually serotonin reuptake (so the brain gets more of the feel-good chemical serotonin) — NEAT movement fights depression from every angle. NEAT activity improves blood circulation through the brain, which sharpens your thinking; it increases the amount of serotonin available to the brain, which improves your mood; and it helps lower stress and anxiety levels, which elevates your general well-being. What's more, while Prozac and its kin suppress your sex drive, regular activity enhances libido, making you happier and more vitally alive.

What's more, a NEAT brain isn't just a happy brain, it's also a healthy brain. A recent four-year study of 749 Italian men and women over age sixty-five found that those who did the most NEAT activity each week, including walking, yard work, gardening, light carpentry, and housework, were nearly 30 percent less likely to develop Alzheimer's disease than those who did the least. And scientists at the Albert Einstein College of Medicine in the Bronx, New York, recently reported that among 469 men and women over age seventy-five, dancing was by far the most effective brain-saving leisure activity, even more so than classic brain builders such as reading, card and board games, and crossword puzzles. According to the five-year review, dancing reduced the risk of dementia by 76 percent, compared to just a 35 percent risk associated with reading. For the healthiest brain, you need both.

NEAT: The True Fountain of Youth

If you could bottle NEAT, it would surely outsell all the antiaging products on the market today, because it actually works! NEAT activity not only increases the quality of your life, but it also actually slows the aging process and indeed lengthens your life.

A study on more than twenty-four hundred twins published in the *Archives of Internal Medicine* found striking differences in the cellular health of those who regularly enjoyed leisure-time NEAT activity compared to those who spent their spare time planted in their seats. The most active men and women showed pronounced slowing of cellular changes associated with aging. In fact, the DNA of the NEAT-living volunteers resembled that of sedentary people a full decade younger. When twins were compared directly, the researchers found that active twins' cells were four years younger than those of more sedentary siblings.

Given these findings, it should come as no surprise that NEAT adds years to your life.

Researchers analyzing data collected from more than five thousand men and women in the Framingham Heart Study found that those who did a regular moderate activity, such as walking, extended their life spans by nearly four years . . . all without breaking a sweat.

NEAT Is the Energy and Quality of Life

It seems like such a small thing, sitting instead of standing. But when a machine is meant to do one thing (stand and walk) and you use it in a completely different way (sitting and sitting), this breakdown is inevitable. This is why you're so utterly wiped out after a single day of sitting in the office, and why you feel so sick and tired over time. Your body is not built to sit ten or more hours a day. In fact, of all the postures you can assume, sitting may be the worst. Even otherwise healthy people can suffer serious health consequences from chair-based living. That's great news for the pharmaceutical industry — Pfizer, the maker of the cholesterol lowering drug Lipitor, pulls down more than $12 billion annually — but grave news for you and I, who pay a terrible price in poor health and empty pocketbooks.

Our bodies and minds desperately want to

stay in motion. When we stop for too long, our systems grow stagnant. Our once-supple arteries stiffen with plaque. Our waistlines bulge, opening the door for diabetes, cancer, and further heart damage. Unused, your muscles atrophy and your calorie-burning metabolism slows to a near standstill, inviting still more burdensome pounds. As the body fails, so does the mind. We sink into depression. So we pop meds, seek comfort in a bowl of nacho chips or Häagen-Dazs, and distract ourselves with hours of surfing the Internet and watching "reality" TV, because this fabricated world is far more enchanting than the one we've created for ourselves. Without movement, there is simply no quality of life.

Indeed, NEAT *is* life. Research shows that walking just 1 mile a day reduces your risk of dying in the next ten years by 46 percent — just 1 mile. There is no greater proof that our bodies are born to move. From the moment we enter this world, our basic biological compulsion is to move. Children are the embodiment of NEAT activity as they wiggle, dance, bounce, swing, and spin in circles until they topple over. As we age, our NEAT declines until we die, which, of course, is the ultimate absence of NEAT. But here's the interesting thing. Though we obviously can't live forever, through NEAT, we can live a lot longer. Instead of accepting a sedentary life that accelerates NEAT decline and, as we are now seeing shortens our life spans through heart disease, diabetes, and other conditions of sitting disease, we can infuse NEAT back into our lives and profoundly prolong life and, more important, quality of life. The Okinawans, the longest-living people on the planet, who routinely live past the one-hundred-year mark, are proof. They don't run marathons or join gyms. Instead, they walk, garden, dance, and move their bodies well into their nineties and beyond.

The NEAT life allows you to live a long life that is buzzing with energy and vibrancy. One in which you aren't worried about your weight or burdened with bad health. One in which your mind is free to dream big. We can turn our lives around. But we must start now. Every day, there are more NEAT-squelching services and devices hitting the market that threaten to steal what little activity is left from our lives. I have proof that NEAT living is within everyone's reach. I have studied people who manage to live a NEAT life despite their sedentary surroundings. I have developed a finely tuned system for helping others do the same. I am confident that everyone can follow in these NEAT footsteps and make sitting disease and its awful consequences a thing of the past. The time is now. Let's get up and go.

2
THIN OR FAT? THE NEAT
DIFFERENCE
"EFFORTLESSLY SLIM" IS EASIER
THAN YOU THINK

You undoubtedly know someone who is infuriatingly trim despite having the appetite of a lumberjack. While you're cutting your M&M's in half, he or she is shoveling down the candy-coated disks by the fistful without gaining an ounce.

Fitness magazines will tell you that your friend has a raging metabolism and if you, too, can't eat pancakes and sausages every morning with impunity then yours must simply be sluggish. That's actually true. Just not in the way you've been led to believe.

Think back to the discussion on mortgage and your metabolism. Remember your basal metabolic rate (BMR), or "metabolism," as people call it, accounts for just 60 percent of your daily calorie burn, and it is largely determined by your size. Just like a big house usually means a bigger mortgage, a bigger body burns more energy. There are some natural variations, but differences in BMR do not account for meaningful differences in weight gain or the ability to eat ice cream sundaes every day. What does is your NEAT metabolism.

THE CASE OF THE MISSING CALORIES

Though the science of NEAT is clear to me now, I stumbled upon it largely by accident (how all great scientific discoveries are made). It happened during a meeting with two renowned colleagues, Dr. Michael Jensen and Dr. Norm Eberhardt, as we were collectively scratching our heads over this exact question: Why is it that some people can completely pig out and not gain an ounce, while others start popping shirt buttons at the mere sight of an all-you-can-eat buffet? Was it possible that those who were overweight just didn't know how much they were eating?

For the longest time, that's exactly what scientists believed. They figured that the people who gained weight simply ate more than they thought and those who stayed slim ate less. But I'm going to tell you something you already know and have probably been frustrated by your entire life. Not everyone gains weight the same way when they eat the same amount of food. Let me say that again, so you can clap your hands and rejoice: You probably don't eat more than you think; and *yes,* your best friend may indeed eat much more than you and still not gain weight. I have conducted the experiments. I have seen the science. In studies where researchers overfeed people in the lab — often by hundreds of calories per day — the differences in weight gain are astonishing . . . and indisputable.

In one such landmark study led by esteemed obesity researcher Dr. Claude Bouchard in 1990, researchers overfed twelve pairs of sedentary male twins (all of them lean with no family history of obesity) 1,000 extra calories a day six days a week (they could eat what they wanted on the seventh) for fourteen weeks. That's 84,000 extra calories over the course of just over three months. He also isolated them in a dormitory and instructed them not to exercise. As you might imagine, everyone gained weight, with the average weight gain being 18 pounds. But the gains ranged from a low of 9 pounds to a high of nearly 30! That's more than a threefold difference. Not surprisingly, the twins tended to be similar in whether they were high or low gainers, which led to speculation about "fat genes." Some people, it seemed, were biologically hardwired for weight gain. It was an interesting theory, but I always suspected that the real culprit behind the scenes was "NEAT genes." If all these people were overeating by such a huge amount yet some were gaining comparatively very little weight, their bodies had to have a system for getting rid of calories. All those missing calories that hadn't been turned to fat had to be going somewhere.

We decided to go on a quest for the missing calories. The first step was conducting our own overfeeding experiment. Fifteen healthy but otherwise sedentary (meaning they didn't "work out") people of all ages and walks of life, including one married couple, stepped up to the plate to volunteer. I threw my own hat in to make it an even sixteen. Then the fun began.

First we built a dream team of one hundred scientists, cooks, dietitians, health professionals, lab techs, and researchers of all kinds to make sure we covered every base — and then some. For the two-month study period, every food item the volunteers ate was hand-prepared by Marty, the head chef, and her crew of five cooks in the kitchen. Each ingredient was weighed to within a gram to ensure we were getting precisely the right amount of excess calories. (Stop reading and skip to the next paragraph if you're squeamish . . . or eating lunch.) To be sure that all those extra calories weren't somehow evacuated in some people, we also had a very admirable team of researchers collecting and analyzing waste (and you thought research science was all glamorous). We spent two weeks carefully monitoring how many calories each needed just to maintain current weight. Then, for the next eight weeks, we stuffed and studied them.

OVEREATING IS GREAT FUN!

During presentations, I can hear people gasp when I tell them we overfed people by 1,000 calories a day. "How is that possible!?" "Weren't they terribly ill?!" they all wonder as though we were fattening them for human foie gras. Truth is, it's incredibly easy, even wonderfully enjoyable to be overfed. That's why so many of us do it daily!

Every day I would come to the lab and set up my experiments. At 9:30, I would go for breakfast, where two fried eggs, often with tiny bits cut off to make the calorie count precise, were waiting for me. There would also be a strawberry milk shake, some apple slices, a small carton of milk, coffee, and a newspaper. Lunch was a large salad with cheese and dressing, ice cream, and often soup. Dinner was a pizza, with crackers, fruit, and a milk shake. It was all delicious and, after feeling a little bloated for the first few days, delightfully easy to get used to.

The only true oddity of this overeating experiment was the spatula. The spatula was used, under Marty's sharp gaze, to have people literally clean their plates and then lick off the spatula. This was not optional, as we had to know that our volunteers were all overeating an extra 1,000 calories on the nose. One night, as I was leaving work, there was an argument going on. Standing there was one of the volunteers, a 6-foot-tall young man. In front of him stood Marty, all 5 feet of her, blocking the exit, saying "you are not leaving until you drink that juice off your plate." This young man was looking down at Marty, belligerently refusing. No one stands down Marty. I watched as this young man lifted the plate to his lips and drank down the juice from the hamburger he had just eaten. He may have stomped off, but he had eaten his extra 1,000 calories — exactly.

The results were nothing short of astonishing. Despite eating the caloric equivalent of an extra Big Mac and large shake each and every day — *56,000 extra calories* over the study period — one volunteer barely gained an ounce. By contrast, another unfortunate lady deposited nearly every extra calorie as body fat and piled on 14 pounds. There was a greater than tenfold variation between extremes. The rest fell somewhere in the middle, with some gaining minimal amounts and others gaining significant pounds. (One fascinating side note is that some of the volunteers who boasted at the start of the study that they could eat anything they wanted and not gain weight gained as much or more weight as those who claimed they piled on pounds with every little transgression.) Myself? I was bang in the middle, having gained a few pounds.

Now we were on to the million-dollar question: How on Earth could some people not gain weight? Where were all those extra calories going? We know that basal metabolic rate, or BMR, the calories you burn simply living and breathing, doesn't change in any meaningful way when you overeat. So they didn't magically fry off the pounds through elevated metabolism. These weren't marathon runners or avid gym goers, so they didn't go out and jog an extra 5 miles or burn it off in boot camp classes. They had to be shedding all these calories through their daily life. But how?

LEVINE MEETS FREDERICK'S

To unlock the mystery, we set about designing "NEAT underwear" (pictured here).

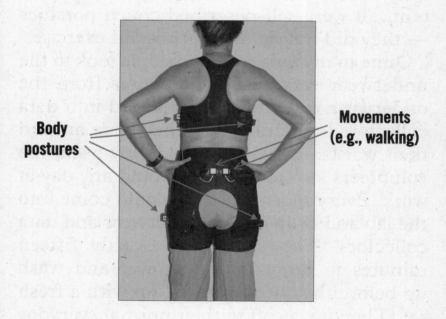

Body postures

Movements (e.g., walking)

As you can see from the photo, they look vaguely like something you'd find at an adult shop on Eighth Avenue in New York, but their purpose is decidedly more functional than fetish. Using technology inspired by NASA, we integrated microsensors into these tank-top- and bike-short-style undergarments, which allowed us to quantify body postures (i.e., sitting, standing, shifting around in a chair) and movements like walking and climbing stairs every half second of the wearer's life. We then recruited twenty intrepid men and women to wear them for ten days straight. Half the group was moderately obese, half was lean, and, most important, all were self-described couch potatoes — they did not do any purposeful exercise.

Quite to my amazement, people took to the underwear very easily. The wires from the underwear were tidied up and fed into data collectors in a fanny pack they wore around their waists. Aside from the fanny pack, the volunteers looked like they would any day at work. Every morning, they would come into the lab and drop off the underwear and data collectors. They then had exactly fifteen minutes to jump in the shower and wash up before they needed to kit up with a fresh set. Then it was off to their normal everyday lives.

At the end of our experiment, we compiled all their data and nearly fried our retinas poring over more than 20 million dizzying data points. It was amazing. Our data analyzer Shelley sat and scrutinized nearly every toe tap. On one occasion, she called me over, concerned. "Look. John got up at three a.m. last night, but only for ten seconds. I wonder if there's something wrong with his setup." We called his wife to check. His setup was fine. Sure enough, he got up in the middle of the night to shut the window. We had that level of detail on peoples' everyday, around-the-clock activity.

To translate all of these movements into calories, we purchased a state-of-the-art calorimeter so that each daily movement was translated into its calorie equivalent. When all these calories were added together, we would have NEAT. After two years of researching, we were ready to find the answer: What is the connection between NEAT and obesity?

As we sat for hour upon hour, translating the NEAT of people as they did everything from hanging Sheetrock to sleeping, a pattern began to appear. It got stronger and stronger until we could barely contain our excitement. It was as though we'd just uncovered the Rosetta stone to deciphering the confounding obesity code.

The difference between the obese men and women and their lean peers came down to one thing and one thing alone: NEAT. Specifically, the obese volunteers sat planted like ferns for a full 2 1/2 hours a day longer than the lean volunteers who stood, walked, and generally fidgeted about that much longer. The math makes perfect sense. When we took the calculations one step further, we determined that if the overweight volunteers in our study adopted the same daily movement patterns of their lean peers, they could burn an additional 350 calories every single day — enough to shed 37 pounds in a year. Bye-bye obesity (which is clinically defined as 30-plus pounds overweight).

To put that in perspective, you would have to take a sixty-minute aerobics class (a full hour of vigorous, sweaty movement) or run (not walk) forty-five minutes every day to burn that many calories. Can you make time to do that? Do you want to? Is it any wonder that exercise doesn't work for so many of us? Society keeps building gyms to help us combat obesity, but the calories we burn behind their mirrored walls pale in comparison to those we could and should be burning in normal life. The healthy, lean volunteers in our study were not gym goers or avid exercisers. They didn't alter their lives to work out at 5 a.m.; they simply lived their life with greater movement, just the way nature intended.

When you consider that the mere act of standing burns three times as many calories an hour as sitting, it all makes perfect sense. If sitting is the problem, standing is the answer. NEAT is the metabolic switch. Those who didn't gain weight in our overfeeding study responded by spontaneously moving more. As they overfed, their NEAT naturally increased. Those who failed to increase their NEAT gobbled through an extra 1,000 calories a day and gained ten times more weight. NEAT is the factor that determines whether you'll get fat when you eat too much (as so many of us do today) or whether you'll remain trim.

SNEAK PEEK BEHIND THE SCIENCE

Shortly after my NEAT research was reported in the *New York Times,* I received an e-mail from a reader challenging me on why on Earth it takes more than one hundred experts and tens of thousands of dollars to conduct this type of study. Understand that when scientific exploration is boiled down to 2 inches of copy on a newspaper page, you don't get much of the setup, just the punch line. But the time, effort, and resources that go into a study like the NEAT obesity paper published in *Science* is no joke. To prepare, design, and carry out this NEAT research, we worked for nearly a decade to bring together all the essential elements.

- Twenty study participants who were willing to forgo Christmas peanut brittle, Halloween Milky Ways, and all restaurant and home meals. Every meal had to be taken at the hospital, without exception.
- A biomedical team of approximately 150 people, including engineers, endocrinologists, dietitians, and specialists to conduct analyses with a mass spectrometer.
- The periodic $1,000 per person glass of water. This was a special metabolic test that required drinking water treated with tracers to monitor the person's metabolism as a way of providing researchers a measure of compliance that test subjects were eating only meals prepared for them by hospital staff.
- A dedicated kitchen staff to cook twenty thousand meals over the test period, starting at 5 a.m. each day —

without skipping a beat, food group, or strange hankering.

- One hundred fifty million lines of data that were downloaded from the data loggers and analyzed.
- Committed study participants who would clean their plates — and scrape them, too — so every calorie that was served was also consumed.
- Custom-made data-logging under-garments that all participants wore twenty-four hours a day, exchanging a new pair every morning at the hospital at breakfast. They had to be ordered to fit a wide variety of body types and be durable enough to stand up to everyday activity.
- Jet fighter control panel motion sensing technology embedded in the special underwear to monitor every tilt and wiggle of the participants.

THE NEAT BEAT

There's a turn of phrase I love: Everyone marches to their own drummer. Nowhere is this more true, or important, than in terms of NEAT calorie burn. Studies show that everyone has a unique NEAT Beat that falls along a spectrum from slow pulsing and down tempo, where their natural tendency is to move very little, to quick and frenetic, where they're always bustling about. As you look around, those men and women who have enviably trim profiles are that way because they manage to march to a steady, consistent NEAT Beat despite an environment relentlessly trying to hold them down.

NEAT ACTIVATOR IN ACTION

Ethan was the one volunteer in our overeating study who didn't gain an ounce. My research assistants were so skeptical that he wasn't "sneaking" in exercise, they nearly took to grilling him under hot lights to make him fess up to what they were sure must be midnight marathons.

Ethan flatly denied doing anything differently in his day-to-day life. He wasn't deliberately deceiving us. It was true that he hadn't become an overnight iron man. But, unbeknownst even to himself, he had started moving more throughout the day. Instead of driving his son to the bus stop as usual, he started walking him there; he got up and paced up and down the sidelines during the boy's soccer games and practices; he was even getting up during the middle of the night to do little things like adjust the drapes and shut the window (he didn't even remember those actions; his wife told us). All these actions — so seemingly insignificant they didn't even register on Ethan's radar — were keeping him from gaining weight despite eating the equivalent of a pint of ice cream every single day.

Ethan was the epitome of a person with a naturally fast NEAT Beat, someone who is naturally hardwired to move in response to food. We're not all so lucky, obviously. But we can all pull a page from his playbook and build NEAT habits that will eventually become second nature.

It's not an all-or-nothing equation, remember. It's a spectrum. At the farthest end of this spectrum are fidgety marathoners, those who can't sit still even when they must be seated and who seek out high levels of exercise to compensate for lost environmental NEAT. There are also "nonexercising" fast NEAT Beaters. They're the ones who find alternative approaches to dissipate NEAT in the face of otherwise sedentary surroundings. They walk to work, pace around the office, go golfing or bird watching on the weekends, and putter around the house at night. (See Neat Activator in Action, above.) At the other end of the spectrum, you have the slow NEAT Beaters who "jump" at any chance to conserve NEAT energy and not move. I once saw a woman driving her car alongside her walking dog in an empty parking lot. I stopped to ask if she was okay or needed help. She smiled and replied, "Oh no. I'm just walking my dog." *That* is an extreme NEAT conservation. Most of us fall somewhere in the middle.

From an evolutionary standpoint, it makes perfect sense to have people fall across all the points of the spectrum. Historically, fast NEAT Beaters were those who responded to famine by slinging quiver and sack across their backs and pressing beyond their usual boundaries in search of food. Their slow-beat peers, on the other hand, would be more inclined to stay home and hold down the fort, conserving energy until rains came, buffalo returned, or their NEAT-activating friends came calling with some exotic dinner. They're not lazy; they are simply following their biological imperative to conserve energy, which in times of scarcity made a great deal of sense. On what part of the spectrum you fall, like everything in life, appears to be the product of both nurture and nature.

NEAT GENES

When people talk about "fat genes," they could be talking about their NEAT genes. Because your propensity to conserve or expend NEAT is wired into your DNA. Or, at the very least, it originates deep within your brain. I know. Thanks to my esteemed colleague Catherine Kotz, who has worked tirelessly studying the NEAT command centers in the brains of rats, I've seen NEAT brain biology up close and in person.

Cathy's research has centered on a brain chemical called orexin. Orexin is responsible for propelling the brain from sleepiness into a state of wakefulness. It originates in the core part of the brain known as the hypothalamus, which is the command central for our most basic biological functions, such as breathing and eating. In her animal studies, she noticed that when she injected orexin into the "feeding" part of the hypothalamus, rats would eat more. Interestingly, they would also move more.

That got us to thinking. What if you injected orexin into the paraventricular nucleus (translation: the part of the brain responsible for basic levels of activity)? Would the animals spontaneously move even more? First, we outfitted twelve rats with tiny skullcaps so we could insert a wire-thin needle into the appropriate part of their brains, (this sounds gruesome; but the rats barely flinch and seem completely unbothered by the process). Then we handed the reins to Lucy, a new young student in the lab.

Every day, Lucy would spend time handling and stroking the rats, so they got used to being picked up and became comfortable with life in the lab. Then the experiment began. In the morning, Lucy would carefully inject each rat with a tiny amount of orexin. Then she placed them back in their chambers, where she would observe them like subjects on reality TV for the next twenty-four hours.

The results were remarkable. Every time orexin was injected, NEAT increased. The more orexin was injected, the more NEAT increased. It was like the rats discovered Starbucks. They would go from lolling about in their pens watching the world go by to darting around the cage, rearing up on their hind legs, polishing their faces with their paws — pure NEAT activities. After about two hours, the orexin would wear off and they'd go back to their usual activity, or lack thereof.

Here's where it gets really interesting. As we were performing our experiments, two other NEAT brain scientists were hot on the trail of an even more compelling finding. Like us, neuroresearchers Colleen Novak and Jennifer Teske found that when you inject orexin into lean, healthy rats, NEAT increases. However, they went a step further and injected orexin into the brains of obese rats. The NEAT response was considerably lower. It was as if their brains were resistant to the effects of the NEAT stimulant. The researchers found the same phenomenon with neuromedin U, another NEAT-stimulating brain chemical. The obese brain showed a dulled response to multiple NEAT promoting signals. As a consequence, obese animals move less and sit more.

To translate this into human terms, it suggests that when the body releases its normal "let's move signal," a person with a slow NEAT Beat, especially one who is overweight, will respond by moving far less than someone with a quicker NEAT Beat. To illustrate the point in real-world terms, here's a snapshot of a day in the life of both.

8:00 a.m. *Each man's wife asks, "Darling, will you go and get the mail on the way to work?"*

- Harry stops at the mailbox in the car as he drives off to work.
- Tim puts on his slippers and dashes to the mailbox despite the cold.

8:55 a.m. *Running late for work.*

- Harry drives as close to the office building as possible and takes the risk of parking in the vice president's doorside spot.
- Tim parks in the very first parking space he sees and races across the parking lot.

11:00 a.m. *Midmorning break.*

- Harry gets coffee from his thermos and calls his wife on his desk phone.
- Tim walks over to the café across the street and calls his wife on his cell phone.

Noon. *Lunch.*

- Harry takes lunch in the cafeteria and chats with a friend.
- Tim grabs a quick sandwich and walks around the building grounds with a friend.

6:30 p.m. *Each man's wife asks, "Honey, will you take the dog out?"*

- Harry opens the back door and nudges the dog out.
- Tim grabs the leash and takes the dog for a walk around the neighborhood.

Both wrap up their day in time for *Monday Night Football*. Harry and Tim each achieved the same end goals. However Harry achieved them with the minimum NEAT and Tim burned many more NEAT calories. Remembering back to our NEAT underwear experiment, it's not difficult to imagine who is overweight and who is lean in this scenario.

Just as we have genetic tendencies for personality traits like stubbornness and altruism and for diseases like diabetes and heart disease, it appears we also have genetic tendencies for our NEAT Beat. But as with the rest of our DNA blueprint, our genetics may load the gun, but the environment pulls the trigger. You are not doomed to a life of obesity simply because you're genetically inclined to conserve NEAT. It simply means you must "cue" your environment with more NEAT stimulators and lower your exposure to NEAT squelchers. Remember, widespread problems with weight are very new in our culture. Our DNA has absolutely not changed in the past thirty years. Our environment has.

As the rising tide of obesity proves, our current sedentary lifestyle and environment have set up a cascade of NEAT-suppressing circumstances that are confounding our most basic biological drives to move, no matter where we fall on the NEAT spectrum. No matter your NEAT Beat, whether you are a NEAT activator or a NEAT conserver, you are now living in a way that is fundamentally at odds with the way your body is hardwired to live. NEAT conservation once served an important function — keeping you alive during times of hardship and famine. Now it simply leads to chair addiction and obesity. NEAT activation once kept us pushing forth into new frontiers — literally. Now we're breaking new frontiers from our chairs, leaving even NEAT activators at risk for overweight and ill health.

THE FIDGET FACTOR

I didn't even want to use the "f word" in this book. But since so many people still consider NEAT as being synonymous with fidgeting, I decided it must be addressed.

As we started to develop the NEAT concept, the world press latched on to one small element of it and deemed it the "Fidget Factor." One headline actually read "Eat All You Want, But Fidget." Other stories encouraged overweight people to tap their feet, twirl their hair, twiddle their thumbs, and even doodle as a way to lose weight. That was never my intent. Yes, every little NEAT motion (and fidgeting is NEAT motion) will give you a little metabolic bump. But these reporters were literally missing the forest for the fidgets.

When we examined the effects of fidgeting in the lab, it was a much broader range of activity than simply scooting around in one's chair. Instead, we asked people to come in and perform their typical home activities in the lab. Some people simply sat on a chair and pressed buttons on a remote control; others folded laundry. One woman even brought in a stuffed cat, which she proceeded to stumble over time and time again (she explained afterward that she actually spent much of her day tripping over the cat!).

You see, NEAT activity included fidgeting,

and, yes, fidgeting is a way that NEAT activators burn off some calories when forced into sedentary situations. But NEAT is more than tapping your toes. It is the movement of life.

NEAT ACTIVATION BEGINS WITH BRAIN CHANGE

Elaine was a self-proclaimed chair addict. Her two-hour daily commute and long hours sitting on the job had robbed her of what little energy she had. She joked that collapsing on her couch each evening to watch TV was her "favorite activity." Besides, she could barely believe that just standing and walking more would provide enough benefit to be worth the effort. But her steadily increasing weight and now nearly constant low back pain were becoming no laughing matter. She started "cuing" her office for more stand-up activity. She placed the reference materials she used several times a day on a higher shelf, forcing her out of her chair every time she reached for one. And she dragged her stationary bike out of the basement and placed it in front of the TV in her rec room, where she pedaled thirty minutes each evening while watching *Seinfeld*.

Slowly, she became more NEAT active all

day, every day. She parked in the far "late-comers" lot at work, though she was one of the first ones through the door. She skipped the elevator and took the winding staircase to her second-floor office. When she got stumped on a project, she got up and took a quick walk around the halls rather than reaching for a snack. After four months, she lost 12 pounds. "Losing weight this way isn't as fast as crash dieting or extreme exercise programs, but I don't mind because I know I can do this for the rest of my life. In fact, now I can't imagine living any other way."

Bingo. NEAT living is about habituation. Breaking old, unhealthy habits — like smoking and sitting all day — and forging new ones. Just as lifelong smokers can crush their Camels once and for all, the most steadfast chair dwellers can literally retrain their brain to prefer movement. Science says so.

Years ago, neuroscientists truly believed you couldn't "teach an old dog new tricks." The brain, they argued, was "set" by the ripe old age of three. After that, you supposedly became more rigid and less open to new experience. During the past decade, however, riveting new brain research has revealed that the adult brain remains remarkably plastic deep into our senior years. In fact, in 1998, Peter Eriksson and his colleagues at

Sweden's Sahlgrenska University Hospital discovered that brains could undergo "neurogenesis" (literally form new brain cells) well into their seventies. More important, the brain's very mode of operation can be remodeled over time, quieting some areas and activating others.

Take what happens in therapy, for example. Someone can be absolutely petrified of spiders and have been since he or she first laid eyes on a eight-legged creepy crawly dangling from the ceiling. Yet through persistent treatment, that person can defuse the brain circuits that go haywire in the presence of spiders and even learn to appreciate the beauty of arachnids. Patterns of brain activity that lead to obsessive-compulsive behavior can be shifted and relaxed. Brain wiring can change. And though it may be easier in youth, it is never too late. Our brain's circuitry does not become indelibly hardwired. What's more, the brain and body are inextricably connected, so what you do physically can have profound mental effects. NEAT activity can help stimulate new cell growth in the brain, making you prone to — you guessed it — more NEAT activity. Like Elaine in the example above, if you change your environment, your brain follows. Before you know it, your brain is leading the way because it has come to expect the behaviors you've been training it to crave.

That's precisely what happened to Penny, who lost 12 pounds while following the NEAT Plan. "I was accustomed to sitting all day with my job. Now if I sit too long, I get fidgety and my legs don't feel right. I have a hard time sitting, which is great, because I don't have to remind myself to get up as often as possible. I automatically do it."

BETTER LIVING THROUGH NEAT

Your ultimate goal is to reengineer NEAT back into your life through both environmental change, tweaking your surroundings to cue NEAT, and through individual change, setting NEAT behavioral goals that will eventually overwrite your chair addiction and become second nature. Exactly how to do that will be the focus of the rest of this book. But it's important to understand that this is a small-step process. Your brain isn't a ball of Play-Doh. It can't be modeled overnight. Rather it takes time, and most important, consistency.

Research suggests that a NEAT behavior that is repeated twenty-one days in a row — that's every single day for about three weeks — will stick. Do it for two months and it's in there for life. The goal is to become addicted to the buzz associated with NEAT. Feeding this buzz as often as you can (at least once daily) will accelerate and strengthen the link your mind makes between motion and increased energy and well-being. This is completely in line with the current thinking in behavioral psychology: "Stimulate early, easily, and often." When my clients falter, it is here at this very first step. They make NEAT harder than it should be.

Like Roberta. She was a lovely lady in her fifties who had been plagued by a persistent weight problem. She became very excited about infusing NEAT into her life and immediately vowed to start running three miles a day, "like I did when I was in my thirties." I tried to talk her out of it to no avail. She lasted six days.

Remember, the difference between obesity and leanness is less than you think. It's *not* hard-core exercise. It's 2 1/2 hours of NEAT improvement. It's two or three walking meetings during your week. It's organizing the toolshed before you watch the game. It's shopping at a mall where you can park in a central location and walk and shop instead of hopping from store to store by car. It's small, consistent steps. It is taking action this very second and repeating that action tomorrow and the next day and the day after that. Through the NEAT Plan, I will show you the way.

3
NEAT MAKEOVERS
SMALL CHANGES EQUAL RADICAL RESULTS

The heart of NEAT is living your life the way you were meant to live it — out of your chair; on your feet; doing things. It's the difference between sitting down, passively letting life pass you by, and getting up and engaging it full steam.

Inevitably, when I explain that to clients, they nod as though they're "getting it," but when I ask, "So what are you going to do differently?" I'm often greeted by blank stares and silence. Most people are sunk so far into their chair-centric lifestyle, they don't know where or how to begin changing it. Many worry that they'll need to upend their entire life to become more NEAT. That's not the case. Instead, it's a series of small adjustments that add up to big life change. It's a lot like climbing a mountain. From afar, the task seems monumental, but each step, from perusing guidebooks to breaking in your boots to taking that first (and second and twentieth) step are very, very doable. It takes planning and commitment, but one day you look up and realize you've reached the summit. It's the same with NEAT. You just start taking steps in the right direction, and in the end, you're living your life, only better.

You'll find a day-by-day plan in the second part of the book. But it will be easier to follow if you get the feel for what an active NEAT life looks like. Here are some examples of NEAT makeovers you can make in your personal and professional life that can have a profound impact on your daily calorie burn as well as your health, happiness, and productivity.

Your NEAT at Work: Invent!

Desk jobs are killing people. If you work outside the house, you absolutely must find ways to get more NEAT at work, because that's likely where you find yourself for increasingly long hours. The statistics are staggering. Almost one-third of office workers are regularly logging fifty or more hours a week. That's a 22 percent increase since 1980. More shocking: The Center for Work-Life Policy recently reported that seventy-hour workweeks have become the new norm for employees hoping to climb their way to the top of the corporate ladder.

Though I'm far removed from the corporate world, I can relate. I frequently pull ten- to fourteen-hour days, which until recently were threatening to kill me slowly. So I'll tell you what I did. I was so disgusted with what sitting twelve hours a day was doing to my health, I went to Sears and plopped down my credit card for a $350 treadmill and a tall drafting desk. With a little creative crafting, I fashioned the two together and created a walking workstation. Now, make no mistake, I wasn't sweating through my suit or gasping and heaving while trying to answer e-mails or converse with colleagues. I only run if there's a fire or I'm chasing a tennis ball. Instead, I set the belt to move at a civilized, very relaxed, sauntering pace — 1 mile per hour.

The results were astonishing. I fully expected to be flagging by late afternoon and utterly wiped out by the end of the day. What actually occurred was the complete opposite. I not only worked more efficiently while on the move, but I arrived home at the end of the day buzzing with energy. NEAT begat NEAT. I scarcely had to plan NEAT into my evening leisure hours because I was vibrating with so much get-up-and-go, I literally went about the house looking for things to do. A shelf to hang here. A closet to remodel there. There was no shortage of home improvements to do, and suddenly I had all the interest and energy in the world to do it.

At the time, I was viewed as an eccentric for my vertical walking workstation. Today, Steelcase is mass manufacturing the Walkstation, a "mobile" workstation on a treadmill that lets you work at the computer, make calls, and do business as usual at an easy, civilized stroll. The company originally thought this workstation would be a "niche" product; they soon came to see it as the future. In our most recent study (which was broadcast around the globe), we asked fifteen overweight and sedentary office workers to give such walking desks a whirl. On average, they boosted their energy expenditure an extra 100 to 150 calories an hour over what they burned working at a conventional desk — enough to shed 45 to 65 pounds in a year if used for even a few hours a day. The best part: After the study was over, the volunteers loved the desks so much they wanted to keep them. After ten minutes adjustment time, they all felt completely comfortable ambling at about 1 to 2 miles per hour while working away — just as nature intended.

I've heard from workers (and even students) around the country who have fashioned their own walking workstations and are reaping the rewards.

- Barbara, a forty-three-year-old telecommunications executive, bought a portable treadmill for her office and started taking all calls on a cordless phone while strolling along at 1 mile per hour.
- Emma, a sixteen-year-old girl who was weary of suffering with obesity, vowed to stroll on her home treadmill while talking to friends in the evening (which, if you know a teenage girl, can add up to *hours* of activity). She graduated high school at 118 pounds and now studies on the treadmill at college.
- Greg, a former Division 1 football player who has worked in health care his entire career, had fallen off of his regular workout schedule, packed on an additional 25 pounds, and was suffering from high blood pressure. He made the decision to take control of his health and started the Gruve program. Between April and September, he lost 18 pounds and reduced his blood pressure from 138/98 to a more healthy 110/68!
- Nat Findlay, the fifty-two-year-old vice president of Canadian operations for

111

Cardinal Health, pulled out all the stops and fashioned a $10,000 custom vertical workstation complete with a $1,500 treadmill. As he told the *Chicago Tribune:* "I was a classic guy on conference calls all day. I'd sit in my chair and have no energy. I thought, 'This is nuts. I'm making a nice salary, but the rest of me is going to hell just sitting there.' At the end of the day, this is what we should be doing. Instead of spending millions of dollars in health care for employees, buy them a treadmill for their desk."

I couldn't have said it better myself. I can hear you now thinking, "Okay, you lost me, Jim. My boss will never buy me a treadmill desk, and heaven knows I'm not making one myself." That's okay. Hopefully, the Walking Workstation will be commonplace in the office of tomorrow, or you might change your mind and give one a whirl as you move through the NEAT Plan. But you can create a more stand-up work environment right now without any special equipment. Here's what you can do.

- Hold walking meetings, where you brainstorm with colleagues on the move.
- Ask your supervisor for a cordless office

phone, so you can stand and pace when taking calls.

- Buy a portable stepper you can use while reading reports and talking on the phone and/or a minicycle to use under your desk while you work. They cost less than $100, and when *Women's Day* asked a group of women to use this type of device just two hours a day (based on my research), the results were phenomenal. One woman lost 4 pounds and 6 inches in a week — more than she had by working with a personal trainer.

As more and more companies are looking for ways to create healthier workforces and insurance companies are offering deeper discounts for companies that encourage their workers to walk and move, you'll likely find that your boss is more willing to help you create a NEAT environment than you might imagine. Here is a mini workday makeover that will leave you more than 30 pounds lighter by the end of one year, even if you do nothing else. (Please note, the calorie figures in the following examples may look low; that is because they're the calories you burn above and beyond your basal metabolism — the calories your body burns just to stay alive. It's the most accurate way to express energy expenditure.)

Your Workday the Old Way

- Morning thirty-minute commute. Drive to the office. Park by your building. Take the elevator to your floor. (15 calories burned)
- Make, return phone calls for an hour in the morning. (15 calories burned)
- Meet in the café for lunch = 45 minutes sitting. (25 calories burned)
- Brainstorming meeting in the afternoon = 60 minutes sitting. (15 calories burned per meeting; 45 for a three-meeting week)
- Take the elevator to the ground floor. Walk to car. Drive home. Equals 40 minutes, mostly sitting. (15 calories burned)

Weekly NEAT total = 395 calories

Too much sitting! Virtually no movement.

Your Workday the NEAT Way

- Park five blocks (one-half mile) from your office building entry. This can be as simple as parking in the lot farthest from your building; parking in another building's lot if you're in an office park, or if you take the subway, get off at the stop before your usual one. Take the stairs to your floor. (80 calories burned)

- Take your calls standing up and pacing. Even if you can't get a stand-up or walking desk, you can arrange your office so you can stand when you talk on the phone. Place a notepad on a bookcase or filing cabinet, so you can take notes without bending down. (100 calories burned for one hour of phone time)
- Punch up your lunch with a thirty-minute stroll, then eat in the café for 15 minutes. (70 calories burned)
- Convert three one-hour sit-down meetings to walking meetings each week. Those project status meetings and brainstormings will run more smoothly (literally) in motion. Just grab your BlackBerry and go. (150 calories burned per meeting; 450 calories burned for three one-hour meetings)
- Take the stairs to the main level of the building. Walk to your car. (80 calories burned)

Weekly NEAT total = 2,100 calories

Now that is NEAT living! I've seen people lose 40 pounds and no longer need their cholesterol meds after just walking farther to work.

Your NEAT at Home: A little DIY Goes a Long Way

For nearly a decade, MTV has entertained us with *MTV Cribs*, an inside look at the luxurious residences of rich and famous hip-hop artists and rock and rollers. It's appropriate that "crib" has become slang for house or apartment, because that's exactly what today's dwellings are — enclosed (often even gated) places where we spend the bulk of our nonworking time, where every whim is practically hand-delivered and where we barely need to move a muscle to get what we want done.

There used to be a popular phrase, "If you want a job done right, you've got to do it yourself." There's actually a lot of truth to that old axiom, and I encourage my clients to adopt it over the "crib" mentality. We've gotten so accustomed to relying on convenience services that we've lost sight of the many advantages there are to a little DIY. For some tasks, you not only get the added benefit of calorie burn, but the job also gets done better and faster. Here's a snapshot of how just a handful can add up.

House and Yard Work the Old Way

- Easy dinner at home means calling for pizza and snacking on chips, surfing the Web, and/or leafing through mail while waiting twenty to thirty minutes for it to arrive. (20 calories burned)
- Cleaning floors is an exercise in waiting for the cleaning service to do it. (2 calories burned)
- Doing laundry is driving clothes back and forth from the dry cleaners. (17 calories burned)
- Weeding flower beds is done by spraying herbicide or calling a lawn service. (10 calories burned)
- Water garden, plants, and grass by turning on automatic sprinkler system. (2 calories burned)
- Letting the dog do his business by opening the back door and checking that the electric fence is activated. (2 calories burned)

Weekly NEAT total = 371 calories

House and Yard Work the NEAT Way

- Easy dinner at home is making a pizza (using a premade pizza shell). Sauté some chicken strips to throw on top and toss together a salad to go with it. (Twenty to thirty minutes; 50 calories burned)

- Tidy up the house by sweeping one room a day. (Fifteen minutes each; 30 calories burned)
- Do laundry by pressing, folding clothes for fifteen minutes a day while catching up on the news. (30 calories burned)
- Keep flower beds sharp by pulling weeds, clipping stray grass, raking out dead leaves and twigs. (Twenty to thirty minutes a day; 50 calories burned)
- Water garden, plants, and grass with a watering can and hose. (Twenty to thirty minutes a week; 50 calories burned)
- Letting the dog do his business by clicking on a leash to walk around the neighborhood. (Thirty minutes a day; 70 calories burned)

Weekly NEAT total = 1,660 calories

For weaving in just 55 minutes of NEAT activity a day for the week, you've burned 1,289 extra calories, enough to shed 20 pounds over the course of a year. Think about that next time you're tempted to pick up the phone or push a button to get the job done.

If you have children, they also provide an excellent opportunity to expend plenty of NEAT playing Frisbee, splashing in the sprinkler, building snowmen, jumping in leaves, planting flowers, and living in the NEAT way children find so natural. String up a badminton or volleyball net in the backyard. Buy a used Ping-Pong table for the rec room. Don't allow inactive play in the house. Even homework can be more NEAT. Who says you have to quiz them on their spelling lessons sitting at a table inside? Go out and quiz them while they jump rope, play hopscotch, or splash in the backyard sprinkler. I know a man who rides a tandem bicycle with his daughter in the park each evening. He puts her homework assignments in a map holder on his handlebar and quizzes her as they pedal down the path (obviously one you can't do on the road; but very clever!).

Like my client Debra, you also can help your children pave the way for their own NEAT life. Debra was a frustrated mom of two preteen boys. Living on a busy street without sidewalks in the D.C. suburbs, there were few places she felt safe walking with her family, though she was easily within "walking distance" of the community swimming pool, the boy's school, shopping centers, and their favorite take-out joints.

For years, she lamented her gridlocked life (and her spreading waistline) until she had a moment of inspiration. Her neighborhood didn't have sidewalks or street trees to protect pedestrians from the constant buzz of high-speed commuters, but the neighborhood just next to her own (which she enviously passed each day in her car) did. She started driving there, parking, and happily walking everywhere else she had to go. At first, the boys griped. But soon they came to enjoy the active start to their day and had an easier time sitting through some of their "boring" classes. Debra enjoyed the fresh air and freedom from her steering wheel. She also enjoyed being able to button the pants she'd given up hope of ever wearing again. "I can't believe I didn't think of it sooner. I get quality time to talk with the boys before and after school. I get some peaceful time for myself. And I still get everything I need to do done."

NEAT in Your Relationships

NEAT is the very movement of life. Once you set the NEAT wheels in motion, there's no limit to how far they'll take you. Every single aspect of your life, from the most monumental to the most mundane, can be hugely transformed with more NEAT.

I find that this is especially true in relationships. When our relationships are no longer vibrant or exciting, we say they've grown "stale." To me that means stagnant, or devoid of the energetic buzz that comes from NEAT. Take marriage, for example. Making a marriage work long term is challenging enough. Trying to keep the "magic alive" when planted 10 feet from the TV in his and her La-Z-Boys is nearly impossible. Here is a snapshot of how more NEAT can help revitalize a marriage.

Marriage "Therapy" the Old Way

- Once-a-week therapy sessions = one hour sitting, listening, talking, sometimes stewing. (20 calories burned)
- Daily "check-in" phone call = six minutes of awkward small talk while at desk at work. (5 calories burned)
- Evening dinner together followed by favorite TV shows = thirty minutes sitting, eating, small talk, and 2 1/2 hours sitting and snacking. (20 calories burned)
- Nightly reading of self-help book = twenty minutes lying down, reading. (3 calories burned)
- Once-weekly perfunctory "relations" =

five minutes. (5 calories burned)

- Weekend "date night" dinner and a movie = three hours sitting, eating, minimal talking. (30 calories burned)

Weekly NEAT total = 241 calories

Too little NEAT burn; too little action and interaction.

Marriage Therapy the NEAT Way

- Once-a-week therapy sessions, followed by walk and talk "recap" = one hour sitting, listening, sometimes stewing; forty-five minutes walking, holding hands, occasionally gesticulating to make a point. (100 calories burned)
- Daily thoughtful gesture: buying flowers from street vendor, making bed, packing the other's lunch = six minutes light activity. (25 calories burned)
- Evening dinner together followed by "improvement project" of choice (each night, one spouse gets to pick something in the house/yard to improve; can be hanging Peg-Board in the garage for the tools or finally digging the nice wineglasses out of storage for display in the kitchen hutch) = 30 minutes sitting, eating, small talk, and

1 1/2 hours light to moderate activity. (70 calories burned)

- Nightly game (board game, puzzle, cards, any fun, interactive, non-TV entertainment) = 1 1/2 hours playtime. (70 calories burned)
- Twice-weekly spirited "relations" = 25 minutes. (25 calories burned)
- Weekend NEAT "date" checking out a new art opening, visiting a museum, having a picnic in the park = 2 1/2 hours meandering, 30 minutes picnicking. (220 calories burned)

Weekly NEAT total = 1,455 calories

You burn an extra 1,224 calories the NEAT way, and have much more fun!

NEAT WITH FRIENDS AND FAMILY

Everyone loves a party. So we find lots of excuses to have them. But as is the case with so much these days, parties tend to be sedentary affairs fueled by too much food. This is especially true of the American favorite: sports gatherings.

It's always struck me as ironic that the culture surrounding sports is so sedentary. It's great fun to watch the game; but we, too, should be involved in the play. Let's take, for example, the granddaddy of all spectator sports — the Super Bowl.

Super Bowl Party the Old Way

- Gather before kickoff for pizza and the big pregame show = three hours sitting, eating, beer drinking. (30 calories burned)
- Watch game = three hours of chicken wings, chips, more beer, and other finger food that sits on the coffee table within an arm's mindless reach, standing occasionally to cheer "Touchdown!" or scream at the ref. (40 calories burned)

Game Day the Old Way: 70 calories

Abysmal NEAT burn.

Super Bowl Party the NEAT Way

- Gather three hours before kickoff. Turn up the pregame show on the outdoor radio and play a game of two-hand touch in the backyard. (Too snowy to run? Bundle up and toss the ball, practicing your Hail Marys.) Run inside for hot chocolate and a snack and head back out for a few more

124

tosses before the game begins. Hang a tire from a tree and offer "house prizes" for whomever can get the most throws through the hole. Equals two hours play, forty-five minutes snacking, fifteen minutes washing up for game. (200 calories burned)

- Set up "sports bar" in a room other than the TV room, where people can go during breaks in the game to grab a drink and a snack = three hours watching game, getting up and down for snacks, standing occasionally to cheer "Touchdown!" or scream at the ref. (70 calories burned)

Game Day the NEAT Way: 270 calories

And that's just one party.

Get the idea? Keep these examples in mind as you move forward in the book. In the next chapter, you'll be creating your own daily NEAT Makeover list. So think of a few ways you can infuse NEAT into your typically sedentary activities to rev your metabolism and get you closer to your health goals.

In many ways, people living in our modern world are like a patient who walked through my doors many moons ago. Jeanie was a twenty-nine-year-old married woman who was about 110 pounds overweight. On the outside, her life looked wonderful. She'd married her high school sweetheart, made a comfortable living, and lived in a nice home. Everything was lovely spare one detail — her husband was abusive. Staring at the soft woven wool cardigan draped across her back as she sobbed before me, pouring out her tragic circumstance, the only words that managed to fall from my lips were "You need to leave." Her head bobbed in agreement.

I picked up the local phone book and looked up "women's shelter" and called the first on the list. They had room for Jeanie. I asked if any of her relatives knew what was going on, and she explained that her mother knew. I then asked if her mom could collect her things, to which she answered that she would get them herself. I responded, "No. You have to go directly there. You cannot go back." She agreed. I validated her parking and gave her $20 for the taxi fare.

Jeanie was on her way.

About two years later, I was standing in line for a cup of coffee at the local mall and felt a tap on my right shoulder. As I turned around, this young, attractive woman with cascading blonde curls grabbed me and hugged me. Now, I should explain that this is not a common experience for me (being grabbed by young women). "You don't recognize me," the young woman said. I didn't. Even when she told me, I still did not remember who she was until she offered to give me my $20 back. Then I remembered. Jeanie. She had left her old life and relocated. She was working as a transcriptionist and taking college courses in the evening to earn an MBA. She was 80 pounds lighter and positively radiant.

I had never counseled her on nutritional recommendations or exercise, yet she had lost 80 pounds. I had not discussed with her behavioral modification, medication, or bariatric surgery. I had not told her to buy a book or read a leaflet. I had not even mentioned the issues of her body weight and its impact on health. Yet there she was, 80 pounds lighter. My only advice to her had been to get up and leave her situation. In so doing, Jeanie had completely redefined who she was, and there was no looking back.

She was no longer an individual who defined herself in the context of being abused. Jeanie's problems and their resolution are intimately related to NEAT. Before she left, she was stuck in a terrible situation, sedentary, and depressed. No one had ever told her it could be different. No one ever told her to get up and go, much less gave her detailed instructions for doing so. She kept up appearances and kept trying to do the right thing. But in the end, she felt broken, tired, and defeated, as so many of us do on a global scale today. It's the product of fighting the natural life force within you. The force that wants you to move. To live to your fullest potential. If Jeanie can find the courage, so can you. Get up. Go!

4

PREPARING FOR
THE NEAT LIFE

LOSING WEIGHT IS ONLY
HALF THE FUN . . .

Where will your feet take you today? That is what I ask each and every one of my clients as they prepare to walk out my office door. It is the central tenet of the NEAT life. It needs to become the central tenet of your life. Where will your feet take you today? It is ultimately up to you.

Be honest with yourself. When you were young, you probably had big dreams. You imagined a life full of vibrancy and action. Maybe you wanted to play in a rock band or be a movie star or travel the world. Whatever your young mind fancied, I'll bet it didn't imagine your grown-up self sitting in endless traffic jams, hunched over a computer all day in a cubicle, or vegging out in front of the television for hours each evening.

When I ask clients to tell me about their dreams, they often look at me strangely and ask what that has to do with weight loss. My answer is everything. Rarely do people want to lose weight just to be thinner or healthier. There's a lifestyle — or, in many cases, an entirely different life — attached to it. When you think of your thinner self, you likely don't just imagine someone in smaller pants. You see a happier, more energetic, more successful person who is doing great, fun things and engaging life to the fullest. The problem is that most people think they must lose the weight first (often through crash dieting), and then they can start "living the life." The NEAT Plan takes the opposite, and infinitely more sustainable, approach. Start living that active dream life *first* and the weight will come off along the way. That is the essence of NEAT — living your life!

The perfect example of this is my client Julia, a successful businesswoman in her mid-forties. She had always been fairly active, but her sedentary office job was starting to take its toll, leaving her with a few extra pounds and less energy than she liked. After six months on the NEAT Plan, she lost 12 percent of her body fat. She's in the best shape of her life, but that's not even the best part. She has pursued her lifelong dream of becoming a jazz singer. "As I was going through my goals, I thought, why haven't I done this yet? So I found a voice coach. She gives me piano pieces that I sing along to in the car. She's even going to help me find good gigs. It's wonderful. And now I also look great in my red dress!" Her story is absolutely brilliant, and one I encourage all my clients to learn from.

This is your one and only life on this earth. What do you want from it? If you're like most of the world-weary men and women who walk through my office doors, your dreams are more modest than the Hollywood fame and riches you longed for in your youth, but no less important and likely more personally fulfilling. Maybe you want to take up photography. Or play tennis again. You want to learn and grow, perhaps take a class. You want to be the one who makes people wonder, "How does she/he do it all?" You want the self-confidence that comes with achieving these dreams. You want the weight loss that comes with living an active, fulfilling life. No matter where you are now, you can get all that and more through NEAT living. You have the goals and dreams. I will get you there. The time is now to get up and go.

YOU HAVE THE POWER; NOW MAKE THE PLAN

You have the power you need to change your life. Every single one of us does. All you need is a plan. Step one is identifying what

131

you want.

Before you do anything else, it's important to put your NEAT Goals in writing. You may be tempted to brush this off, but it's a vitally important step. Physically writing down your dreams for the future forces you to think about them in concrete terms, to literally define what you want from life and put it in black and white. Plus, the act of writing your goals is a NEAT activity. So it's the perfect place to start.

There are no limits to what you can dream or how many goals you can have, but make them as well defined as possible. For instance, if one of your NEAT Goals is "I want more energy," take it a step further and say what for, as in "I want to have more energy to ride bikes with my kids in the evenings." If you want to feel better about yourself, say why: "I want to enjoy (rather than dread) shopping for clothes with my friends." Now give it a try. Take out a notebook and fill in the following sentence: In my dream life, I _____. You can fill out as few or as many lines as you wish. But you must fill in at least one NEAT Goal. Write your number one NEAT Goal here:

GREEN-LIGHT YOUR NEAT GOALS

Now it's time to plan how you're going to

132

make your NEAT Goals a reality. That means finding room for and activating NEAT in your life. Remember, the difference between being lean, healthy, and energetic and being dragged down by excess weight, fatigue, and sitting disease is a little over two hours of NEAT activity a day. Yes, I am asking you to create space for 135 minutes of NEAT each and every day. Before you toss the book to the floor in disgust, it's not as difficult as you think. When done properly, NEAT doesn't take time away from your life; it fits within your life. Indeed, it gives you *more* time to live your life. It's the freedom to get out of your chair and go live your life to the fullest. And let's face it: There are 1,440 minutes in a day; you deserve 10 percent of those, which is all the NEAT Plan adds up to — 10 percent of your day. Surely you deserve 10 percent of your day for yourself and your life's goals.

Think about how you currently live your life and spend your day. Ask yourself some hard questions about how you use your time and energy.

How many hours is your television on each day?

How many shows do you watch each evening?

Do you hire a lawn care and/or cleaning service?

Do you drive from store to store when they're less than eight blocks from each other?

Do you drive anywhere a mile or less away?

Do most of your leisure-time activities entail sitting, eating, and/or drinking?

How many hours a day (outside of work) do you surf the Internet?

How many nights a week do you eat take-out, delivery, or drive-through?

How many meals a week do you eat out?

How many extracurricular activities do you take your kids to each week? _____ Do you sit during them?

Do you routinely take the elevator to go less than three floors?

How many hours a day do you sit at work?

How many hours a day do you spend sitting down?

Be honest as you answer these questions. They're not meant to shame you. They're meant to show you how easy it is to be very inactive even if you don't intend to be that way. And when you start filling out the NEAT activation charts that follow, you'll know exactly where to start to change that.

NEAT ACTIVATOR IN ACTION

Lisa already had a hectic life as a mom of one toddler and the co-owner of a successful midsized business. Then she had twins. "I looked at my life and thought, 'There is no more room. I can't fit in another single thing,'" recalled Lisa. "The only way I was possibly going to exercise was to work it into my life, especially into my job where I spend so much of my time."

Inspired by a news story I did on the Walkstation treadmill desk I mentioned earlier, Lisa had a handy friend of hers fashion a desktop to her treadmill. She got on it a couple hours a day to make calls and check her e-mail. The pounds started coming off. Inspired, she searched for more places to put NEAT in her life. "I had an elliptical trainer at home I never used because it seemed like so much effort to change clothes and get all sweaty and have to shower," she recalls. "Then it dawned on me that you're burning calories whether you're strolling along or working up a sweat. It all counts! Now I step on with my regular clothes when I want to go through the mail or catch up on the news. It's so much better for me than sitting, and I don't have to do anything special to get activity in my life. Plus, when I'm walking around or on the elliptical, I'm not snacking. So I save hundreds of calories a day."

Lisa has hit her goal weight of sub-140 pounds following the NEAT plan, but she's had another revelation. "The weight loss isn't the biggest benefit," she said. "I feel so much better. I don't have all those lulls in my day where I'm just fatigued and looking for food or caffeine to lift me up. I'm so energetic now. I've been able to make all these little changes without changing my life. It's freeing to know exercise can be so easy."

Now I'd like you to dig out your personal planner, PDA, or whatever you use for your daily calendar. The first step to making room for NEAT is getting a clear picture of how you're spending your time. On the following pages, you will find two charts: One is a typical weekday; the other a typical weekend (or nonworkday). Fill out each, being completely honest. Sometimes patients feel ashamed to admit they watch two or three hours of television at night or kick back and veg to a full day of football on the weekends. But again, this self-evaluation is not about shame. It's about empowerment. It's about making positive change in your life. It's also not for anyone's eyes but your own. So turn off your filter and write the plain facts. You have nothing to lose but weight.

You'll find two main columns, time and activity, to record what you're typically doing at any given time of day. Under the activity column are three additional columns, indicating the NEAT activity level. List your activity under the appropriate column, depending on how active it is. Any task that is completely idle should fall under Sitting/Inactive; those that require standing or light activity go under Standing, and those that have you on your feet and on the go belong under Moving. I like to take this exercise a step further with my clients and have them mark each activity with the colors of a stoplight. For instance: Take a green marker (or one of your kids' crayons) and make a green dot by the moving activities; make a yellow dot by the standing activities; and put a red dot by the sitting/inactive activities. Red is a color we naturally associate with negative things (like all those red pen marks on school papers), so seeing a lot of red can help shock some people into action. Likewise, we associate green with everything "going" as it should, so it's very satisfying to see an abundance of green marks.

MOVE IN A NEAT DIRECTION

Review your daily activities on the schedules from the preceding pages. Now decide which ones you can "move in a NEAT direction" by making more active. Look especially hard at the red, sitting activities. These are the big NEAT squelchers that lead to sitting disease. You want to change those at least to yellow, but preferably all the way to green. Take, for example, Melanie, an employee in a hectic human resources company. Her daily activity sheet was one big flat red line of sitting. Many of her daily tasks were inescapably chairbound, but others could be "NEAT activated." As part of her NEAT Plan, she identified the items on her daily roster that she thought she could actually do better standing or on the move. Not surprising, her "thinking tasks," like brainstorming and strategic planning, topped the list. She started getting up with pen and paper to walk

A DAY IN YOUR LIFE (WEEKDAY)

Time	Activity	Sitting/ Inactive	Standing	Moving
5:00 a.m.				
5:30				
6:00				
6:30				
7:00				
7:30				
8:00				
8:30				

A DAY IN YOUR LIFE (WEEKDAY)

Time	Activity	Sitting/ Inactive	Standing	Moving
9:00				
9:30				
10:00				
10:30				
11:00				
11:30				
Noon				
12:30 p.m.				

A DAY IN YOUR LIFE (WEEKDAY)

Time	Activity	Sitting/ Inactive	Standing	Moving
1:00				
1:30				
2:00				
2:30				
3:00				
3:30				
4:00				
4:30				

A DAY IN YOUR LIFE (WEEKDAY)

Time	Activity	Sitting/Inactive	Standing	Moving
5:00				
5:30				
6:00				
6:30				
7:00				
7:30				
8:00				
8:30				

A DAY IN YOUR LIFE (WEEKDAY)

Time	Activity	Sitting/Inactive	Standing	Moving
9:00				
9:30				
10:00				
10:30				
11:00				
11:30				
Midnight				

A DAY IN YOUR LIFE (WEEKEND)

Time	Activity	Sitting/Inactive	Standing	Moving
5:00 a.m.	_____			
5:30	_____			
6:00	_____			
6:30	_____			
7:00	_____			
7:30	_____			
8:00	_____			
8:30	_____			

A DAY IN YOUR LIFE (WEEKEND)

Time	Activity	Sitting/Inactive	Standing	Moving
9:00	_____	_____	_____	_____
9:30	_____	_____	_____	_____
10:00	_____	_____	_____	_____
10:30	_____	_____	_____	_____
11:00	_____	_____	_____	_____
11:30	_____	_____	_____	_____
Noon	_____	_____	_____	_____
12:30 p.m.	_____	_____	_____	_____

A DAY IN YOUR LIFE (WEEKEND)

Time	Activity	Sitting/Inactive	Standing	Moving
1:00				
1:30				
2:00				
2:30				
3:00				
3:30				
4:00				
4:30				

146

A DAY IN YOUR LIFE (WEEKEND)

Time	Activity	Sitting/ Inactive	Standing	Moving
5:00				
5:30				
6:00				
6:30				
7:00				
7:30				
8:00				
8:30				

A DAY IN YOUR LIFE (WEEKEND)

Time	Activity	Sitting/ Inactive	Standing	Moving
9:00	_____	___	___	___
9:30	_____	___	___	___
10:00	_____	___	___	___
10:30	_____	___	___	___
11:00	_____	___	___	___
11:30	_____		___	___
Midnight	_____	___	___	___

and think and jot down her ideas. When she needed to brainstorm with a colleague, they did so on the move, walking around the city square outside their corporate headquarters. Suddenly, she had an easy hour or two of NEAT activity every day. She lost 5 pounds in three weeks without changing another thing in her life.

THE MYSTERY OF THE OVERWEIGHT MAILMAN

"If NEAT is the answer to obesity, then why is my mail carrier overweight?" an inquisitive reporter once asked me. It's a good question, and perhaps one you've been pondering yourself. Indeed, though most of us spend our days seated, there are still those, like mail carriers and restaurant servers, who spend long stretches on their feet. How is it they could be overweight?

The answer is twofold. One simple possibility is that their fueling is out of line with their NEAT activity. As you will see in the next chapter, when and how you fuel is an important part of the NEAT equation and can certainly contribute to weight loss or gain. By following a few simple NEAT fueling rules, these active workers would most certainly lose weight. Another essential element to the NEAT life (and weight loss) is self-fulfillment, plotting your goals, and achieving your dreams.

For many, many of my clients, weight gain is a by-product of feeling unfulfilled in life. When you're dissatisfied, your overall energy levels drop, and you likely eat more without even being aware that you're eating. When you start moving toward your goals and improving your satisfaction with life, your energy levels rise, and the weight comes off. I have had patients lose nearly 100 pounds without me ever so much as mentioning physical activity or diet. I simply ask what they want from their life and help them take the first few steps toward their goals. Then they get up and live themselves lean. It's truly amazing, and par for the course in the NEAT life.

Now go through the same mental process. What currently sedentary activities can be NEAT activated? Telephone calls are often the easiest for my clients. Instead of sitting at your desk making return phone calls sporadically, assign specific times of the day to make calls — say, 10:30 a.m. and 3:00 p.m. Then get up with your cell phone and do it on the move. If you have a BlackBerry, you can do the same thing with e-mails (just be careful not to bump into anyone or to do this while crossing the street). As a bonus, this helps structure your day and manage your time, so you're not constantly interrupted by calls and e-mails. Once they "get" the concept of NEAT, my clients also discover the joys of their unused exercise equipment. Like John, who began our conversation by telling me, "I'm not really willing to change much." He wanted to lose about 20 pounds, but had no desire to change his eating habits (his job requires courting potential clients over food for breakfast, lunch, dinner, drinks, etc.). A lightbulb went off once he learned the importance of NEAT activity.

"It was eye opening for me to realize there are ways to do the things I normally do but in a more active way," he said. "Instead of just watching the game in front of the TV on the couch, I can do it on my treadmill, which I never use because I always thought, 'Treadmills are for running and "exercise."' But you can just get up there and walk comfortably and get hours of activity. It's changed the way I think about things."

Or there was Anna, a stay-at-home mom of two, whose every waking second seemed to be sucked up by shuttling her kids to activities and then sitting and waiting for them to be done. It was a moment of sheer liberation for her to realize she could use her kids' active time for her own NEAT activity. She started rambling around the fields while they played T-ball and soccer. She strolled outside and made calls during dance class. She even started practicing their sports and dance moves with them on weekends! And she lost 20 pounds doing it.

THE POWER OF PLANNING

My client Paul epitomizes the power of specific NEAT target planning. Instead of saying, "I will walk an hour more every day," as many do, he identified specific walking opportunities in his day and pinned his NEAT goals to them. Here was his simple, yet brilliant NEAT Plan.

"I always watch CNN for thirty minutes before going to work, so I am going to put the treadmill in front of the TV and watch CNN walking on the treadmill at 1.5 miles per hour for half an hour before having my shower in the morning. On Monday, Tuesday, and Friday, I meet my boss for forty minutes and he has agreed to switch those meetings to 'walk-and-talk' meetings. I have a few favorite shows I like to watch each evening, so I will walk for sixty minutes while I watch."

That was his plan. And it worked. This transition was completely painless for him. He never had to think about when to walk; it was on his schedule. He lost weight and improved his health without carving an extra second out of his day to "exercise."

Now go back to the schedule pages and put an arrow by the activities you can do in a more NEAT way. Instead of meeting a friend for dinner and drinks, plan to go window-shopping. Walk the dog down the block and back instead of just letting him in the yard for ten minutes. Even the smallest activity counts. Identify at least three activities to NEAT activate from your weekday and weekend schedule. But don't go overboard. If you try to change too much at once, you'll get overwhelmed. Keep it simple and doable. Write them down in the chart that follows. Then link your makeovers to your NEAT Goals. Earmark this page, so you can refer to it once you get to the NEAT Plan and need to start adding NEAT activities every day.

MY DAILY NEAT MAKEOVERS

My Old Way

Watching the Sunday game on the sofa

Drive my son to the bus stop

Phone calls sitting

1. _____

2. _____

3. _____

4. _____

My New (NEAT) Way

Walk on treadmill for the second half

Walk him there

Phone calls standing and pacing

1. _____

2. _____

3. _____

4. _____

I am one step closer to my NEAT Goal(s) of

_____

Stumped on ways to work more NEAT into your daily life? Sometimes it helps to consider the "NEAT tools" you may already have at your disposal. These are pieces of equipment or technology that can help you do an otherwise sedentary task on the go. Here are a few of my favorites.

Cell phone. It has all the numbers you need right at your fingertips, so you can catch up with all your contacts while strolling around the house, office, or downtown.

Cordless phone. You never need to talk to someone sitting down again. If you're in your office or cube at work, just stand up and stretch while you talk. Pace, if possible.

BlackBerry. Now you don't even need to be glued to your computer to take care of your e-mail. Stand, stroll, and text.

Any unused cardio equipment. No need to change clothes, get sweaty, or ever feel uncomfortable. Just climb aboard and move at a natural, invigorating pace as you go through your junk mail catalogs, watch your favorite shows, talk on your cell phone, and so on. You're limited only by your imagination.

iPod. Love to read? Great. Reading is a wonderful NEAT activity, and you should continue enjoying the written word. At the same time, you also can download a few podcasts or tunes and enjoy them while you take a walk.

Moleskine (mol-a-skeen-a) notebooks. These pocket-size notepads have recorded the musings of great minds since van Gogh and Hemingway. Of course, it doesn't have to be a Moleskine brand; any portable pad will do. The point is to have a handheld notebook that gives you the freedom to create your to-do lists, outline projects, and do other thinking work on your feet.

Digital voice recorder. Maybe you think better out loud than on paper. Grab one of these amazingly light devices and chat into it as you walk. Most of them plug right into your computer, so you can download your ideas.

Video game console. What? Video games? Active? You bet. Trade your sofa-based gaming system for a Wii, which you actually have to move to work the game. Try popular games, such as Guitar Hero and Dance Dance Revolution, which make you get up and move for active playtime with your kids.

Dog. Not a piece of equipment, but you know where this one is going. If you have a dog, you have the greatest excuse to get out more. Your canine companion needs NEAT, too.

Stability ball. These large inflated balls are perfect "chairs." They encourage you to bounce and stretch and move while you're seated. Plop one by your home computer and/or in the TV room.

Stretch bands. Tie a few elastic stretch bands around your office and/or home desk. Grab the ends and work your arms while you're waiting for Web pages to download.

YOUR NEAT TOOLBOX

Now create your own NEAT toolbox. Write down ten items for your personal kit.

1. _____ 6. _____

2. _____ 7. _____

3. _____ 8. _____

4. _____ 9. _____

5. _____ 10. _____

As you go through the NEAT Plan in the next part, you will be given explicit NEAT instructions — active "to-dos" for the day. Many of these will call upon specific NEAT tools from your NEAT toolbox. (I may also recommend investing in some special, easily affordable, NEAT devices.) So don't feel as though you have to set your entire NEAT course in this chapter. The goal here is for you to start laying the mental groundwork for NEAT living. Start looking at your surroundings and the household and workplace tasks you do differently. I want you to get a vivid picture of how NEAT will blow through your life, energizing it, without disrupting it.

What's the Big Deal?

I'm not much of a betting man, but if I were, I would wager that right about now you're thinking, "What difference is this going to make? I've tried a million exercise programs. How is this going to do anything different for me?"

Go back to the chart on pages 139–148. Look at how much movement has been engineered out of your life. Look at the crushing effect it's had on your metabolism. If sitting is the problem, standing is the answer. Moving is even better. To make the enormous power of NEAT as concrete as possible, I've created the NEAT Burn Chart.

Because determining the calorie burn of individual activities is an inexact science that depends on a host of variables from how much you weigh to how vigorously (or not) you're moving, and because I have found that my patients never actually count calories, especially when the numbers are hard to add up (e.g., 62 + 27 + 103 . . . forget it), I've decided to make it easy for you by breaking down activities into red, yellow, and green calorie-burn categories. Red activities are extremely sedentary, such as lounging and watching TV, and burn just 0 to 50 calories per hour. Yellow activities generally have you up on your feet and puttering about. Activities such as standing and stretching while on the phone and chopping vegetables for dinner fall in this category. A few of the more energetic sitting activities, such as board games (e.g., Cranium), crafts, and sewing, also fall into yellow. They burn 50 to 100 calories per hour. Green activities have you on the move and include things such as mowing the lawn and playing with your kids. They burn 100 to 200 calories an hour.

Notice how easy it is to burn a lot of calories over the course of a day when you choose mostly green and yellow activities. This is the NEAT difference. You have the opportunity to make dozens of active decisions each and every day. Every decision boosts or suppresses your NEAT burn. Every calorie boost brings you closer to achieving your NEAT Goals. When you learn about your calorie burn for specific activities, it becomes very easy to plan your NEAT day. For example, I now know that pushing my mower around my yard for 60 minutes burns approximately 215 calories above my BMR.

NEAT ACTIVITY	CALORIE BURN CATEGORY		
Home Activity	Red (0–50/hr)	Yellow (50–100/hr)	Green (100–200/hr)
Barbecuing/grilling		X	
Cleaning (picking up clutter, etc.)			X
Clearing out storage space/garage			X
Cooking dinner		X	
Grocery shopping			X
Hanging pictures			X
Ironing		X	
Laundry			X
Organizing closets			X
Painting walls			X
Redecorating (moving furniture)			X
Sweeping			X
Vacuuming			X

Yard Activity	Red (0–50/hr)	Yellow (50–100/hr)	Green (100–200/hr)
Fetch with dog			X
Gardening (digging/ mulching/planting)			X
Mowing lawn			X
Planting flowers			X
Pruning shrubs			X

	Red (0–50/hr)	Yellow (50–100/hr)	Green (100–200/hr)
Raking leaves			X
Shoveling snow			X
Trimming hedges			X
Washing car			X
Watering plants			X
Weeding			X

Hobbies, Recreation	Red (0–50/hr)	Yellow (50–100/hr)	Green (100–200/hr)
Baking (e.g., bread, cookies from scratch)		X	
Bicycling			X
Bird watching			X
Board/card games		X	
Bowling		X	
Dancing			X
Fishing			X
Frisbee/outdoor games			X
Hiking			X
Journaling (while strolling)			X
Knitting/sewing		X	
Kayaking			X
Piano/musical instrument playing		X	
Reading (lounging)	X		
Reading (standing)		X	
Skiing			X
Surfing the Web (sitting)	X		
Surfing the Web (standing)		X	

	Red	Yellow	Green
Swimming			X
Tai chi			X
Tennis			X
TV watching	X		
TV watching on elliptical trainer			X
TV watching on stationary bike			X
TV watching on treadmill			X
Video games (seated)	X		
Video games (Wii or moving style)			X
Volunteer work (setting up/serving meals)			X
Window-shopping			X
Yoga practice			X

General NEAT Movement	Red (0–50/hr)	Yellow (50–100/hr)	Green (100–200/hr)
Climbing stairs			X
Pacing			X
Pushing stroller			X
Riding in a car	X		
Standing and talking		X	
Stretch band exercises		X	
Stretching		X	
Walking (strolling pace)			X
Walking and talking (briskly)			X

Walking around the home/office	X
Walking the dog	X
Walking to work	X

As the NEAT wave continues to grow, so does the technology to support it. For those who love to have the newest gadgets, there is the Gruve. Newly released from a company aptly named Muve, the Gruve is a postage-stamp-sized device you wear on your waist via a thin elastic strap. It reads every single footstep and hip wiggle, keeping constant tabs on your NEAT calorie burn, so you always know how much you've moved.

THE NEAT JOURNEY — TRULY THE ROAD LESS TAKEN

"I don't have time!" That's the biggest, loudest protest I hear from the hundreds of harried clients I treat each year. But once they embark on their NEAT journey, they realize that it's not a matter of carving out any more time, but rather using the time they have and doing the tasks of daily living in a more NEAT way.

Laura, a working mother of three young kids who has been shedding a pound a week since starting to live NEAT, described it best: "I've made it my goal to be 'less energy efficient.' I take the stairs when I can. I read the paper on my stationary bike. If I'm craving a snack, I take a walk first to see if I'm actually hungry or just nervous or bored. I not only feel more energetic, but I feel like I'm setting a good example for my kids." Now it's your turn. Start moving in the NEAT direction today.

5
How to Fuel Your NEAT Life

MOVE, EARN, EAT . . . AND LOSE!

Dieting makes you overweight. That was the conclusion of a most intriguing letter to the editor in the *British Journal of Nutrition* a few years back. In it, the author, G. Cannon, explained that those who diet often lose weight in the short term, but over time they usually gain it back and quite often end up weighing more than they did before they started — a phenomenon with which most dieters are sadly familiar. Cannon believed this "rebounding" effect was actually an evolutionary mechanism to protect us from starvation during times of famine. After a period of food deprivation (i.e., the diet of the month), your body may actually ramp up its hunger signals to drive you to eat beyond your normal desired amount and stow away those excess calories as fat in anticipation of the next period of food deprivation. Hence, the more you diet, the more you may end up weighing.

I can't say with scientific certainty that dieting packs on pounds, but I do know this: Dieting in and of itself does not work. Deep down, you know it, too. If it did, we would all be thin, and we wouldn't need any more diets. But each year ushers in a new crop of "eat this, not that" plans promising to put us back into our skinny pants. Am I saying that what you eat has no bearing on your ultimate weight? Most certainly not! Your diet — the food you fuel yourself with day in and day out — is fully half of the weight-loss equation. But it only works if you pair it with the other half: NEAT, the energy of life. Before you turn the page to embark on the NEAT Plan, it's important to understand how you're going to fuel the trip.

As you'll soon see, I have developed a fuel plan to live by, which is carefully crafted to give you the energy you need when you need it most. The plan includes general rules for NEAT fueling, daily fueling tips, and a day-by-day fuel plan that looks a lot like a "diet," but is meant to be a guide for fueling NEAT. The plan is designed to give you an intimate understanding of how the food you eat fuels the activity you do throughout the day. You'll eat more when you need a bigger "fuel cell" to keep the furnaces firing, and less when you're only doing a bit of activity. Though you will certainly lose weight through NEAT alone, you will see results faster if you know how many NEAT fuel cells you really need each day.

USE MORE NEAT ENERGY, LOSE MORE WEIGHT

In a society where food has become a form of entertainment, it's easy to forget that every bite you eat is really a form of energy. You and every living and nonliving thing that moves requires energy to keep going (like the Energizer Bunny!). Consider your car. It needs fuel to run. Since you always need a little gas in the tank for short trips and emergency situations, you never let the gauge hit empty. When it's time to drive longer distances, you top off the tank with more fuel. That's energy balance. And it's exactly how NEAT eating works.

Now, I'm sure you've bought a diet book in the past (or at least leafed through one), and I bet your eyes started to glaze over right about the point where the authors started talking about "calories in and calories out" and calorie-balance. Though calories are important, we're not going to talk about them here; and I don't want you obsessing over the whole calorie balance notion. Here's why. When you get in your car, what is your objective? Is it to balance your gas intake with the miles you drive? Sure, you may try to drive a fuel-efficient car and aim to get good gas mileage, but never in a thousand car journeys is energy balance your objective when you get in the car. You get in the car to go places and do things! It is exactly the same with your body. You don't wake up each morning and say, "Today I'm going to match my calories in with my calories out!" That's never a daily objective. Your objective is to do things, to reach your goals, and to thrive in your life. You eat along the way to keep yourself energized to reach these goals. That is the essence of true, meaningful energy balance — your NEAT driving your food intake, so you are literally fueling your movement day in and day out. The problem is that most of us are so out of balance that we have completely lost sight of the purpose of food and what it does for our bodies. That's why I tell my clients to think of every morsel they eat as "potential energy."

Think back to your ninth-grade Newtonian physics. Remember the apple falling from the tree? That's potential energy changing to kinetic energy. Energy exists in many forms. It cannot be created or destroyed. So it simply changes forms. It's like a battery inside a toy car. The chemical energy is stored inside the battery. When you turn the toy car on, the chemical energy is transferred to the electric motor of the car, and the car obtains kinetic energy and moves.

To lose weight and maintain weight loss, you must learn to link your energy intake (via food) to your NEAT. A simple equation to work by is move-earn-eat. Once you start moving, you set in motion a cycle of replacing your spent energy to keep you in motion. Most people who come into my office with weight problems have this equation in reverse. They start by restricting food to the point that they drain their tank to zero. As if it's not bad enough that they've been sitting all day, they now have absolutely no potential energy. Their NEAT is completely suppressed and their metabolism all but grinds to a halt. Client after client complains that he or she is eating next to nothing, yet the scale won't budge. Indeed, in Britain, obesity rates have doubled since the 1980s, yet energy intake appears to have actually *decreased.* In many cases, people who are obese are actually eating far less than their lean peers.

On the flip side of this equation are those who routinely overfill their tanks without burning off the fuel. Going back to the car analogy, this is similar to walking out to the drive, gas can in hand, and pouring gasoline into your car (and subsequently all over the driveway) despite the fact that the tank is full and you're not driving anywhere today. Now, instead of having no potential energy, you have more than you'll ever use. Putting too much energy in storage results in weight gain, which, in excess, can suppress NEAT by making it difficult to put your body in motion. People who overfill their tanks, like those who let them run dry, are also out of touch with the move-earn-eat equation.

The good news is that NEAT works for everyone on the spectrum by systematically linking activity to food intake and food storage. The simple fact of weight gain is that the body can only gain fat or energy stores if you take in more fuel than you use. Likewise, you cannot lose stored energy or fat unless you burn off more fuel than you take in.

CLEAN FUEL FOR NEAT ENERGY

There aren't any forbidden foods in the NEAT diet. But most of my clients find that the NEAT plan works best when they fill up on natural, nutritionally balanced foods rather than empty calories from overly processed sugary foods or too many heavy, high-calorie foods.

As Christine, a forty-year-old mother of two young boys explained: "Even though I was running regularly, I had a hard time maintaining a healthy weight because I was constantly filling up on sugary foods. I would go for a run, but then I would have jelly-filled doughnuts for dinner. I would burn through those sugary treats quickly and then my energy would fade, leaving me wanting to snack more to get more energy. My eating and energy were all over the map and completely out of whack." Once she started the NEAT Plan, she moved more all day and started fueling more in tune with her activity. "Now I'll have an apple or a yogurt, which keeps me going with steady, even energy that I use as I walk throughout the day. I naturally have more energy. So when I do run, I'm able to make smart food choices to refuel when I'm done, instead of craving a quick sugar fix."

Keep this in mind when making your food choices and select foods that are satisfying, yet bring just the right amount of fuel into your body. That means eating fewer foods that pack a lot of calories per bite, because they're more likely to overfill your tank, and focusing on foods that contain fewer calories per bite but still fill you up, like fruits and vegetables. Combining both strategies is a proven recipe for weight loss. In a recent study published in the *American Journal of Clinical Nutrition,* men and women who strove to include large helpings of fresh fruits and vegetables in their diets lost 33 percent more weight after six months than those who focused on cutting fat alone. I see that in practice every day.

Not surprising, your best source of balanced energy sources is the earth. Foods that come from nature and that have undergone very little processing (i.e., they haven't been stripped of nutrients or had sugar, preservatives, and chemicals added in) tend to contain a healthful mix of carbohydrate, protein, and fat, as well as essential nutrients like vitamins, minerals, and antioxidants that your body uses to function.

Which brings me to fast food. Fourteen percent of Americans eat a diet that consists almost entirely of fast food, according to a report released by Mintel, a consumer intelligence research company. Young adults eat even more, with 22 percent of this group fueling themselves on a diet comprised of mostly fast food, convenience food, and frozen dinners. Fast food is a NEAT enemy. It not only tends to be calorie dense and nutritionally barren, but also it takes absolutely no energy to obtain it. So you expend virtually zero NEAT feeding yourself food that is bursting with energy (which is therefore sure to go straight to storage). In one fifteen-year study of more than three thousand young adults, those who ate fast food more than twice a week gained about 10 pounds more than those who ate it less than once a week. It's that powerful.

I recognize the need for fast food once in a while, but truly only once in a while. Though it seems like a bargain to feed a family of four for $25 in less than ten minutes, the real cost is astronomical when you consider the price you pay for health care and prescription medications for poor nutrition and weight-related ailments such as high blood pressure, diabetes, and high cholesterol. For the same $20 to $30, you can feed your family wonderful, real food that doesn't take all that long to cook. Chicken breasts can be sliced and sautéed, tossed with some lettuce, sprinkled with cheese and salsa, and wrapped in a tortilla for a cheap, healthy meal in less than fifteen minutes. With a little preparation, you can have hard-boiled eggs, baked potatoes, baby carrots, and sandwiches ready to grab and go when you need to put food on the table quickly.

I also recommend having one or two nights a week where you eat "slow food."

Take a little time to cook something nice, even if it's just for yourself. Make it a fully NEAT experience — chopping, kneading, folding, stirring, and savoring the process of preparing, cooking, and eating whole food such as lean meats, grains, fruits, and vegetables. Before you can fully connect your eating to your NEAT, you need to fully connect to your food. It's difficult to feel a true connection to a greasy foil-wrapped burger and oil-stained cardboard container of fries some kid tossed through your open window while you riffled through your pockets for change. It's easy to appreciate and connect to a beautiful, savory meal you've prepared for yourself. And you expend NEAT making it. A true win-win. And it's all built into the NEAT Plan.

SNACK ATTACK!

Snacking is supposed to be a way to avoid overeating by quelling your between-meal hunger pangs so you don't overdo it once you sit down to eat. A recent food and health survey shows that 93 percent of Americans eat at least one snack a day. The problem is, many of us are now overeating our snacks. Some experts estimate that we get about 25 percent of our daily calories through snacks. That wouldn't be a problem if we ate a little less at meals and were snacking on fruits or nuts. But for most Americans, snack time is 500 additional calories piled on top of meals, and these calories come in the form of vending-machine potato chips, candy bars, or cookies or a rich, creamy coffee concoction. Your NEAT eats will allow for the snacks of your choice, but I beg you to choose wisely. Treat those Cheetos and nachos like fast food — okay once in a while, but not everyday fare.

THE EIGHT RULES FOR NEAT FUELING

NEAT fueling will help you lose weight if that's your goal. But it's about much more than dropping dress or pants sizes. It's about living vibrantly, free from fatigue and diet-related disease. It's living life the way it's meant to be lived. You must follow these NEAT fueling rules whether or not you have pounds to lose.

1. **If you don't recognize it, don't eat it.**
    Simple enough. The best foods were

once growing in nature. If what you're about to eat is so processed that it is un-recognizable as food that has come from a natural source, it shouldn't be on your plate.

2. **Eat breakfast every day.** Your morning meal primes your NEAT engine. It does not have to be a lumberjack special (in-deed, unless you're chopping trees for a living, it should not be), but it is not optional. Interestingly, in a recent survey, 90 percent of men and women name breakfast as the most important meal of the day, while only 49 percent report eat-ing this meal seven days a week. Break-fast skipping has a direct connection to weight gain, because it leads to overeat-ing and subsequent fat storage later on. It has no part in the NEAT life.

3. **Breakfast must include fruit.** Breakfast is so essential to NEAT eating that it oc-cupies two slots on the list of rules. Fruit contains disease-fighting antioxidants and energy-boosting natural sugars that help inspire NEAT activity. You must eat some every morning.

4. **Lunch and dinner must include a fruit or a vegetable.** Remember our discus-sion of fuel economy and how fruits and vegetables are ideal nutrient-dense,

177

low-energy fuel sources? That's why they are essential to include in every meal, including lunch (where they're often over-looked) — they provide essential nutri-ents while filling your stomach with fiber, so you're less likely to overeat more calorie-dense foods such as cheese and bread.

5. **Slow-Food Wednesdays.** The fast-food habit can be hard to break, especially if it has become a way of life. By designat-ing one day a week as fast-food free, you force yourself to explore your options. Once you do, you'll find alternatives that are so much tastier and leave you feeling so much clearer and more ener-gized, you'll soon be driving right by the drive-through most days each week.

6. **Fat-free Fridays.** Pledge to yourself not to eat fatty foods on Fridays. By fatty, I don't mean salmon or fatty fish, of course. I mean cookies, cakes, fried foods, and other unhealthy fats. I know this is a tall order for many people who like to "let loose" at the end of the week. But I chose this day intentionally. If you can stand your ground and make wise food choices (try the shrimp cocktail) during high-temptation times such as happy hour, staying committed to the

tenets of NEAT eating other times will be effortless.

7. **No eating in the car.** Nothing good was ever eaten behind the steering wheel (or in the passenger seat) of a moving vehicle. It's a bad habit and not in line with NEAT living. Designate your car a food-free zone.

8. **Cook something on Sunday.** Sunday dinner used to be a nearly sacred tradition in the American household. Though it has been steadily replaced by sporting events and other extracurricular activities, Sunday is still the perfect day to visit the local farmers' market and/or grocery store to stock up on food to cook, if not for the evening, than for the week ahead (I like to do both!). Make a soup or stew that you can freeze in portable containers and take to work. Roast chicken and potatoes. Cook a batch of hard-boiled eggs. An hour or two of NEAT cooking on Sunday will reward you with easy NEAT eating all week long.

The NEAT Fuel Cell System for Weight Loss

Ultimately, move-earn-eat should be as natural as brushing your teeth in the morning — you'll just do it without giving it a second thought. But if you've lived the better part of your life dieting on and off or eating mindlessly without any thought to activity it may take a while to make the connection. That's why I've developed the NEAT Fuel Cell System.

As the name implies, fuel cells represent energy to burn. You want to take in and burn the right amount of fuel to power your journey day in and day out. With fuel cells, I've taken out the guesswork and done the calculations for you.

Each fuel cell is worth 200 calories. You start with seven fuel cells each day. Most of your meals will be two fuel cells. Snacks will be one. Fruits and vegetables are free and can be consumed with abandon. You may find yourself craving food if you're used to mindlessly eating, but if you spread out your fuel cells throughout the day, you should not actually be hungry. Because too much change at once is a recipe for failure, you will be adopting the fuel cell system gradually during the plan, starting with breakfast and working through lunch and dinner and finally to snacks.

Fuel Cell Guide

Here is a guide to give you a concrete idea of the fuel cell value of commonly eaten foods. As a reminder, one fuel cell equals 200 calories. You get seven fuel cells a day on the NEAT Plan, and all fruits and vegetables are free (meaning you don't have to count them toward your fuel cell quota; eat as many as you'd like). Once you get a feel for how much fuel your favorite foods provide, you will no longer need the chart. It will become second nature, just like NEAT. Note: I did not include vegetables and fruits, since they are free. Also, though I always prefer that patients eat fresh food over packaged, there are a number of healthy frozen foods on the market today that work perfectly with the NEAT fuel plan (since they tend to be 350 calorie meals). Feel free to incorporate those as needed.

BEANS, PEAS, AND SOY FOODS

Food	Serving	Fuel Cells
Beans (black, pinto, etc.)	1/2 cup	1/2 fuel cell
Chickpeas	1/2 cup	1/2 fuel cell
French beans	1/2 cup	1/2 fuel cell
Green peas	1 cup	1/2 fuel cell
Lentils	1/2 cup	1/2 fuel cell
Snap beans	1 cup	1/2 fuel cell
Tempeh	3/4 cup	1 fuel cell
Tofu, firm	1/2 block	1 fuel cell
Tofu, regular	1/2 block	1 fuel cell

BEVERAGES

Food	Serving	Fuel Cells
Apple juice	8 oz	1/2 fuel cell
Cocoa	8 oz	1 fuel cell
Coffee, black	6 oz	0 fuel cell
Cola	1 can	1 fuel cell
Cranberry juice	8 oz	1/2 fuel cell
Grapefruit juice	8 oz	1/2 fuel cell
Grape juice	8 oz	1 fuel cell
Lemonade	8 oz	1/2 fuel cell
Lemon-lime soda	1 can	1 fuel cell
Orange juice	8 oz	1/2 fuel cell
Tea, brewed	6 oz	0 fuel cell
Tonic water	1 can	1/2 fuel cell
Vegetable juice	6 oz	1/2 fuel cell

BREADS

Food	Serving	Fuel Cells
Bagel	3 oz	1 fuel cell
Bread	1 slice	1/2 fuel cell
Cornbread	1 small slice	1/2 fuel cell
English muffin w/jam	1 regular	1 fuel cell
Muffin	3 oz, small	1 fuel cell
Pita bread	1 pocket	1/2 fuel cell
Roll or bun	1 small	1/2 fuel cell
Roll or bun	1 large	1 fuel cell

CONDIMENTS AND SPREADS

Food	Serving	Fuel Cells
Cream cheese	1 oz	1/2 fuel cell
Honey	2 tbsp	1/2 fuel cell
Hummus (regular recipe)	1/3 cup	1 fuel cell
Jam/jelly	2 tbsp	1/2 fuel cell
Ketchup	1 tbsp	0 fuel cell
Maple syrup	2 tbsp	1/2 fuel cell
Margarine	2 tsp	1/2 fuel cell
Mayonnaise	1 tbsp	1/2 fuel cell
Mustard	1 tbsp	0 fuel cell
Pickles	1 oz	0 fuel cell
Salad dressing, full fat	2 tbsp	1 fuel cell

DAIRY PRODUCTS AND EGGS

Food	Serving	Fuel Cells
Cheese	1 oz	1/2 fuel cell
Cottage cheese	1/2 cup	1/2 fuel cell
Eggs	2	1 fuel cell
Milk	8 oz low fat	1/2 fuel cell
Yogurt	8 oz nonfat	1/2 fuel cell

DESSERTS AND SWEETS

Food	Serving	Fuel Cells
Brownie	1 small 3/4 oz	1/2 fuel cell
Caramel candy	1 oz	1/2 fuel cell

Cheesecake	1 2–3 oz slice	1 fuel cell
Chocolate	1 1/2 oz	1 fuel cell
Coffee cake	2 oz	1 fuel cell
Cookies	4 small	1 fuel cell
Doughnut, plain	1	1 fuel cell
Frozen yogurt, nonfat	1/2 cup	1/2 fuel cell
Fruit pie	1 slice	1 1/2 fuel cells
Ice cream, scoop	1/2 cup	1 fuel cell
Ice cream, soft serve	1/2 cup	1 fuel cell
Jelly beans	10 (1 oz)	1/2 fuel cell
Pudding, chocolate	1/2 cup	1 fuel cell

FAST FOOD

Food	Serving	Fuel Cells
Burger, cheese	1 small	1 1/2 fuel cells
Burrito, bean	1	1 fuel cell
Cheesesteak	9 oz	2 1/2 fuel cells
Enchilada, cheese	1	1 1/2 fuel cells
French fries	20–25	1 fuel cell
Fried chicken	2 drumsticks	2 fuel cells
Pizza, meat and veggie	1 slice	1 fuel cell

FISH AND SHELLFISH

Food	Serving	Fuel Cells
Bass	3 oz	1/2 fuel cell
Catfish	3 oz	1 fuel cell
Clams, small	20	1/2 fuel cell

Cod	3 oz	1/2 fuel cell
Crab, Alaskan King	3 oz	1/2 fuel cell
Flounder	3 oz	1/2 fuel cell
Lobster	3 oz	1/2 fuel cell
Mahimahi	3 oz	1/2 fuel cell
Salmon, canned	3 oz	1/2 fuel cell
Salmon, sockeye	3 oz	1 fuel cell
Scallops, large	4	1/2 fuel cell
Shrimp, steamed	3 oz	1/2 fuel cell
Tuna, canned in water	3 oz	1/2 fuel cell
Tuna, fresh	3 oz	1 fuel cell

GRAINS AND PASTA

Food	Serving	Fuel Cells
Couscous	1/2 cup	1/2 fuel cell
Macaroni	1 cup	1 fuel cell
Oatmeal	3/4 cup	1/2 fuel cell
Pasta	1 cup	1 fuel cell
Rice, brown	1/2 cup	1/2 fuel cell
Rice, white	1/2 cup	1/2 fuel cell
Soba noodles	1 cup	1/2 fuel cell

MEAT AND POULTRY

Food	Serving	Fuel Cells
Bacon	3 slices	1/2 fuel cell
Beef, ground	3 oz	1 fuel cell
Beef, ribs	3 oz	1 1/2 fuel cells

Beef, steak	3 oz	1 fuel cell
Buffalo, steak	3 oz	1/2 fuel cell
Chicken breast	3 oz	1 fuel cell
Chicken thigh	1	1/2 fuel cell
Goat	3 oz	1/2 fuel cell
Ham, deli	2 slices	1/2 fuel cell
Hot dog, beef	1	1 fuel cell
Hot dog, turkey	1	1/2 fuel cell
Knockwurst	1 link	1 fuel cell
Lamb, chops/leg	3 oz	1 fuel cell
Pastrami, beef	2 slices	1 fuel cell
Sausage, Italian	1 link	1 fuel cell
Turkey, breast	3 oz	1 fuel cell
Turkey, deli	4 slices	1/2 fuel cell

NUTS AND SEEDS

Food	Serving	Fuel Cells
Almonds	1 oz	1 fuel cell
Brazil nuts	1 oz	1 fuel cell
Cashews	1 oz	1 fuel cell
Macadamia nuts	1 oz	1 fuel cell
Peanut butter	2 tbsp	1 fuel cell
Peanuts	1 oz	1 fuel cell
Pecans	1 oz	1 fuel cell
Pistachios	1 oz	1 fuel cell
Sunflower seeds	1 oz	1 fuel cell
Walnuts	1 oz	1 fuel cell

Oftentimes my patients ask if they can follow their regular diet, such as Weight Watchers or a physician-prescribed nutrition plan, while also following the NEAT Plan. So long as it is a nutritionally sound program, like Weight Watchers is, I say absolutely. Do keep in mind the Eight Rules for NEAT Fueling, however. By always eating breakfast, filling up on fresh fruits and vegetables, limiting fast food, and spreading your calories evenly throughout the day, you will get more mileage from any diet plan you follow.

DEFINE YOUR NEAT FUELING MATRIX

When you fuel up is nearly as important as what you fuel up with. Again, the ultimate goal is to use food as fuel for NEAT activity, so steady, predictable fueling is a must. As mentioned, you will be starting with seven fuel cells a day. You can use them on the foods you like, but I recommend portioning them out, for example, in three two-fuel-cell meals and one one-fuel-cell snack, so you have a steady stream of energy all day, which also helps you avoid overeating.

When many of my clients walk through the door, their fueling patterns are either completely haphazard, with them mindlessly eating small bits of food, which never satisfy them for any meaningful stretch of time throughout the day, or, worse, they don't eat all day and pile on the food from 6 p.m. to bedtime.

Both of these methods — grazing all day without giving a second thought to what, when, or why you're eating or starving yourself all day only to empty the fridge at night — are incompatible with NEAT fueling and make meaningful weight loss slow and difficult.

For satisfying, lasting energy, it is far better to eat three solid fuel cell meals. Or, if you are a snacker by nature, lighten up two of your meals, and redistribute those fuel cells in two daily snacks when you need them most. Remember fruits and vegetables are always free, however; so if you eat an apple at 10 a.m. and a bunch of grapes at 3 p.m., *they don't count toward your fuel cell allotment.* Think about how you prefer to eat, taking into consideration what time you rise, take work breaks, get home, and finally go to bed. Distribute your fuel cells to provide a satisfying, steady flow of energy throughout the day.

Even the simplest beverages today — such as coffee — can be loaded with potential energy (calories!). Check out the fuel cell value of these popular Starbucks drinks and choose wisely next time you pony up for a pick-me-up.

Café Americano	0 fuel cells
Café au Lait, w/whole milk	1 fuel cell
Café Latte, w/nonfat milk	1 fuel cell
Cappuccino	1 fuel cell
Cappuccino, w/ low-fat milk	1 fuel cell
Caramel Frappuccino Coffee — no whip	1 1/2 fuel cells
Caramel Frappuccino Coffee — whip	2 fuel cells
Caramel Macchiato	1 1/2 fuel cells
Coffee Frappuccino Coffee	1 1/2 fuel cells
Mocha Malt Frappuccino Coffee — whip	3 fuel cells

6

Kicking Off the NEAT Life: A Step-by-Step Plan to the Body and Life You Want

I want you to imagine something for a moment. Imagine living a life free from the burdens of extra weight, one in which you don't fear the doctor's office, because your blood pressure, cholesterol, and blood sugar are all in check. One in which you're free from the burdens of self-doubt and the feeling that life is passing you by. Imagine a life in which you come home in the evening brimming with energy instead of sapped and spent. Imagine walking through your neighborhood and seeing families playing in their yards, kids riding bikes, and parks filled with young children playing.

That is the NEAT life. It's how things used to be before we became trapped by sedentary living. Before kids began holing up inside and sitting utterly motionless in front of video screens for hours on end. Before we started living virtually on our seats rather than experiencing real life on our feet. It's how things need to be again if we hope to return to health and wellness.

In case you're skeptical, convinced such a way of life is a relic of the bygone past, I assure you there are places today where the NEAT life is alive and thriving. They are called Blue Zones, places on the planet where scientists have found people living exceptionally long, healthy lives, such as Okinawa, Japan, which I mentioned earlier, as well as Sardinia, Italy, and Loma Linda, California. Residents of these places commonly live past one hundred and suffer a fraction of the diseases that plague people in other parts of the developed world. What do they have in common? Constant, moderate physical activity that is an inseparable part of their daily life. Social activity. And a plant-based diet. Sounds a lot like NEAT living, doesn't it? That's because it is!

Your NEAT Life Starts NOW

You are about to embark on a journey that will change your life. It's about so much more than losing weight (though that will happen). It's about breaking free from the rigid, stifling confines of modern life and daring to stand up, stretch your expectations, and question the status quo. It's about being accountable to yourself for the quality of your life. Instead of mindlessly sitting for hours blearily staring at your computer screen while you down your sixth cup of coffee for the day, you'll be on your feet, engaged and active. Instead of plopping down in front of the TV in the evening wondering where all your energy went, you'll be buzzing with activity. It's a journey that if taken properly has no end, but only becomes richer and more expansive the farther along you go. It will not, however, all be easy.

The NEAT Plan is a life change. It will take forethought, preparation, and true commitment. This book is your guide. The plan in the pages that follow is your map. I am your sherpa. During the next eight weeks, I will lead you every single step of the way as you learn the ropes. Some of the steps may seem odd, and there will be many twists and turns. You may falter or feel like quitting. But there is a method to what may sometimes seem like madness. Each step you take and task you complete is scientifically designed to make you think, feel, and live in a more NEAT way. As you move through the plan and take on the NEAT life, those tasks that once seemed so odd will begin to make sense. The to-dos that originally felt forced will become second nature. You will develop a completely different approach to traditional "eating and exercising" that is at once simple and profound. You will lose weight, gain energy, and, most important, acquire knowledge and skills that will carry you through the rest of your NEAT life. I predict that by the time you turn the last page of the plan, you will take the torch from me and pass it along to a friend or loved one. You yourself will become the sherpa. In fact, I encourage you to reach out from the start and include your spouse, children, friends, and loved ones on this journey. Shared experience is the ultimate in NEAT living.

A DAY IN THE NEAT LIFE

Each day for the next eight weeks, you will be assigned specific NEAT tasks. Some of these tasks you will perform just once; others will be repeated day after day. Together, they will help you reach your NEAT burn goal for the day and set the stage for permanent life change. They will be divided into three categories: NEAT Feet, NEAT Beat, and NEAT Fuel Cells.

NEAT Feet

Walking is the heart and soul of NEAT living. By replacing one hour of sitting with one hour of even the most gentle, easy-paced walking, you burn an extra 100 to 200 calories per day. At the end of a year, that simple one hour per day adds up to more than 20 pounds — without going to a gym, without changing your clothes, and without breaking a sweat. When you walk more purposefully, you burn more and lose more — still with no gym or sweat towel required. The basic bottom line is that the person who walks the most, burns the most. We have walked for 7 million years; it cannot be a surprise that this is how we are meant to function.

Take it from Connie, a mother of seven, who started walking two hours a day on the treadmill while making calls and performing other tasks. "I lost eleven pounds and 10 percent body fat," she said. "The best part is I'm so much healthier and more energetic. I didn't get sick once this winter. I'm not falling asleep during my hour-long commute. Walking is easy; people just forget to do it. Every night after dinner, our family takes our dogs for a forty-minute walk. It's just part of our day. My husband walks instead of taking the cart when he plays golf. When we go to hockey games, we walk around the concourse between periods rather than just sitting there. At first, we had to consciously plan our walking; now we just do it. Movement is a priority in our lives."

That's why you'll receive a NEAT Feet prescription that starts at three twenty-minute walks every day. *This is not optional.* Whenever possible, strive for three separate walks each day instead of walking for a full hour in the morning and sitting the rest of the day. You cannot get up and walk on your treadmill as you watch your favorite morning show (though that *is* a great way to start the day) and then park yourself virtually motionless in a chair for the next twelve hours and consider yourself living a NEAT life. For the best results, you need the repeated spikes in NEAT metabolism throughout the day. You will also find a few exercises that will help condition your body for NEAT activity.

I'll confess that if you currently live a chairbound existence, these daily walks may feel disruptive at first, as you will need to find a way to schedule them. Eventually, as you integrate walking into your typical daily activities, they become practically seamless. For instance, while working on this book, my coauthor, Selene Yeager, and I would often meet to brainstorm. We could have easily sat in a café and chatted for an hour or two over food and drinks. Instead, we grabbed notepads and pens and walked about town. It was a brilliant way to do business. We not only accumulated hours of NEAT, but the flow of ideas was faster, and the ideas themselves were better, when our bodies and brains were on the move.

Ideally, NEAT Feet activities should take place on your feet. But if along this journey you fall madly in love with riding a bike or swimming at the Y, I'm not going to discourage you. Any activity in which you are moving your body can count toward your NEAT Feet quota. That includes (but is not limited to) activities such as:

Aerobics classes or DVDs
Cooking classes
Cycling
Dancing
Gardening
Golfing (sans cart)
Home and yard work
Martial arts
Playing outdoor games with your kids
Singing lessons
Skiing
Swimming
Tennis
Visiting art gallery
Yoga class

Throughout the plan, you will also find an assortment of exercises that can help you get up and get NEAT throughout what might be an otherwise sedentary day.

No matter what other activities you do, at least one of your daily NEAT Feet bouts should take place on your feet, using your legs to carry your body weight. Your NEAT Beat activities should be similarly standing and walking based.

NEAT Beat

NEAT Beats are activities designed to turn up your natural NEAT rhythm, which, though especially important for those with slower NEAT Beats, is essential for everyone living in today's NEAT-suppressing world. Some of these activities may seem strange or even frivolous. But do not discount them. They have been crafted around scientifically grounded and long-established psychological principals that are crucial for sustaining NEAT and health in the long term.

One of the first things you'll notice is that though many of the NEAT Beats are physical actions, such as going to a museum, others are mental exercises that involve planning and dreaming, such as drawing a picture that represents your goals. Science teaches us that the brain is biologically driven to need NEAT. It is the active pulse of our life, like our heartbeat. The NEAT Beats are designed to feed your brain's cravings for

NEAT and in turn the brain will start thinking and behaving in a more NEAT way. For change to truly stick, you need to think differently. By creating a new mind-set, you can create new routines, and before you know it you have a whole new lifestyle. Not everyone is comfortable with creativity and self-expression, so some of these tasks may be challenging, but try to embrace them as an opportunity to grow. And remember, many of these NEAT Beats have you up and moving, so they count toward your NEAT Feet prescription for the day.

"I really liked the mental exercises," said Ken, a thirty-four-year-old father of two, who lost 26 pounds and 7.5 percent body fat on the NEAT Plan. "I'm not a great artist, but I liked drawing my ideal life. I drew a picture of my family and I taking a walk and being active. It was an awakening for me. The things I enjoy most — dancing with my wife and playing with my kids — also ended up being the biggest calorie burners. You don't have to join a gym or go on some special diet. Just making these little changes to live a more active life makes a huge difference. The positive effects have spilled into the rest of my life; I even acted on my dream to write a book."

Ken's story is a perfect example of how

each NEAT Beat is like a stone splashing in a pond. As it hits the surface, the ripples send energy throughout the water. That's how it works in your life. At the end of eight weeks, the cumulative affect of your NEAT Beats should be like a sonic boom that causes your life to buzz with unstoppable energy that literally rocks your world. When you are through with this program, it is the NEAT Beats that will resonate most in your life as you continue to live your life in a completely new, healthy, vibrant way.

NEAT Fuel Cells

As you saw in the previous chapter, NEAT fueling is not about systematically denying yourself food or subsisting off of some special powdered-drink mix. It is about linking your NEAT burn with your fuel intake, just as nature intended. I developed the NEAT Fuel Cell System and the Eight Rules for NEAT Fueling to make it easy.

Since bad food habits can be even harder to break than sedentary living, I designed the NEAT Eat part of the plan to be progressive. You'll start by transforming breakfast — the most essential fuel of the day — and gradually work your way through the rest of the day's meals and snacks until you are eating your seven fuel cells a day every day. Because

I don't want you to become a slave to counting calories, I have included clear descriptions in chapter 5 of how many fuel cells the most commonly eaten foods contain. By the end of the program, you should be able to eyeball a plate of food and give a pretty accurate guess as to its fuel cell count.

Some people ask me if following the eating plan is necessary for weight loss. As I mentioned earlier, the answer is no. If you do more than infuse more NEAT in your life, you will lose weight. The catch is that most people want to lose weight quickly. If your eating is very out of sync with your NEAT activity (as most people's is), it will take longer to lose weight through NEAT activity alone. By following the NEAT Fuel Cell System, you can easily speed your weight loss and likely lose more weight overall. Even if you have no weight to lose and/or choose not to adhere to the fuel cell system, you must still follow the Eight Rules for NEAT Fueling. These are designed to feed your body clean, nutritious fuel that builds healthy muscles, bones, and immunity and enhances NEAT living and activity.

NEAT REWARDS

Rewards. Everyone loves them. You likely have at least one credit card in your wallet that rewards you for spending money, and any number of punch cards from coffee shops, delis, and other local businesses that reward you for frequenting their shops. Well, adopting a NEAT lifestyle is more important than any mocha latte or random purchase, so I feel you should reward yourself as you hit important milestones along your journey.

These rewards are called NEAT Treats, and they will be awarded using a point system based on your NEAT activity. Each day will be assigned a certain number of points based on your NEAT Feet, Beat, and Fuel Cell prescriptions. Some days your NEAT Beats will be more involved, so they'll be assigned more points; other days they'll be easier and assigned fewer. Every two weeks during the program, you'll be able to award yourself a NEAT Treat if you reach a certain number of points. Let's say, for instance, the maximum number of points you can earn during the first two weeks is 90. You don't have to be perfect to get rewarded, just consistent, which means scoring at least 75 percent of your potential points for that two-week period. Score 68 or more points and you earn your first NEAT Treat.

As is the NEAT way, you will be determining your own NEAT Treats. They can be something as simple as a new CD or something as elaborate as a Caribbean Cruise. But they should be progressive in that the first NEAT Treat is relatively small and the final, fourth NEAT Treat is quite meaningful. Emily, a fifty-year-old bookkeeper who lost 20 pounds using the NEAT system, rewarded herself along the way with gardening tools to support her favorite NEAT activity. Her first NEAT Treat was a pair of gardening gloves. Her second NEAT Treat was a padded garden caddy so she could work on her knees with greater comfort. And so on. None of her Treats was particularly expensive, but each made her happy and reaffirmed her commitment and enjoyment of NEAT activity.

How would you like to reward yourself for your successes on the NEAT journey? Make your NEAT Treat list right now.

1. _____
2. _____
3. _____
4. _____

CONTRACT WITH SELF

Before the start of each two-week period, you'll find a Contract of Commitment. It helps clients stay on track and push through tough times when they put their intentions in writing and commit — in ink — to a contract with themselves.

If you feel unsure about signing this contract, you may not be prepared to embark on the NEAT journey. Sure, you want to lose weight and feel more energetic. Everyone does. But you can't succeed without commitment. And I don't mean commitment to me. I mean commitment to yourself. Commitment to taking the time you need to reach your goals. If you're feeling uncertain, you're likely still in the contemplative stages of change. That's perfectly okay. I encourage you to go ahead and read the book without following the plan. You will learn a lot along the way and may be inspired to make some positive life changes. You can always come back to the book and follow the plan when you're ready. Readiness cannot be rushed. But by continuing to explore and contemplate, you will steadily and more quickly move toward the starting line.

THE SEVEN TENETS OF THE NEAT JOURNEY

NEAT is the energy of life. Indeed it is life. As you start your NEAT journey, there are some principles I would like you to keep in mind and take to heart.

Invent. The ultimate creation is the human — that is you. You are unlimited in your potential. You are so powerful that you are able to change your own life. Every week starts with creation.

Worship. You have to believe in something. Whether it is a deity, nature, or some collective human spirit, it is crucial to recognize that there is something beyond you. Whatever your approach to understanding the world, embrace it once a week.

Invest. Invest of yourself and judge others with generosity. It will change the way you look at the world. Instead of feeling closed down and afraid of the world, you will embrace it with energy and enjoyment. Your generosity will ripple out to others and ultimately back to you. Be generous. Be humble. Be kind.

Live. Your mind, body, and spirit are yours. How you live is up to you. Many of us don't have all the advantages or money to do exactly what we want every day. But you do have the ability to choose how you want to live every day.

Love. Love is the greatest part of the human experience. Tell your kids you love them. Find ways to love your work. Love your friends. Every person you encounter should be improved by your interaction. Give love fearlessly without worrying about what you will (or will not) get in return.

Do. There is a simple bottom line to the NEAT life. It is DO! Do great things — think later. Go now, take that step toward your dreams and goals. When in doubt, do it now!

Offer yourself. If others had not shared a kind word, a few bucks, mentorship, or opportunities with you, would you be where you are today? Find someone to share your life's successes with; by sharing your successes, you raise others to a higher plane.

■■■■

Part 2
The Plan

■■■■

7
WEEK 1: PLANTING THE SEEDS OF CHANGE

Week 1 is devoted to sowing the seeds of NEAT change. As excited as you may be to dive right in and get going, it's important to get off on the right foot if you want this life change to stick. Too often I see clients catapulting themselves into the middle of the journey rather than starting at the beginning. By bypassing those essential early steps, they end up quickly overwhelmed and throw in the towel shortly after they begin. I won't let that happen to you. Instead, we're going to take this week to lay a solid foundation. The NEAT Feet prescriptions will kick off with a base level of walking; your NEAT Beats will literally set the tone for the eight weeks (and beyond) to come; and the NEAT Fuel Cells will help you start each day right with — what else? — your morning meal.

Ready? Let's begin.

This is a two-week commitment to myself. I am ready to commit two hours per day to my NEAT plan. Some of the steps along the way may be challenging, but I will do them. I know I am on a new journey and that there may be twists and turns. Sometimes I will stumble — but I will always get up. Sometimes I will want to give up — but I won't.

I am ready to change: _____

Day 1: Monday

NEAT FEET: Three twenty-minute walks

There's a saying in art and design circles: Form follows function. If an instrument needs to perform a certain task, it must be designed in a way that allows it to do so successfully. That is to say, your body is built to walk, so your life should be formed in a way that allows you to do that. That's NEAT living, as you know; and the ultimate goal is for these walks to slide seamlessly into your day while you are doing other things. But if you're used to working and living from a chair, it will take some practice to make that happen. Don't wait until you figure out how to work in your walks; go out and get started immediately. Take a notepad and pen with you, and jot down tasks you can do on the move. Then, next time you walk, include one of those tasks.

NEAT BEAT: Buy a plant

Your first NEAT Beat is to buy a plant that is less than 6 inches tall that you can keep in a prominent place like your desktop or on a counter in your home where you will see it frequently. You are probably thinking, "What is this? A plant? What does a plant have to do with losing weight or getting in shape?" The plant is iconic of the NEAT journey we will take together. It will need to be nurtured and watered and cared for to thrive and grow. Neglect it, and it will wither away. Your plant should serve as a constant reminder that you are a living organism that needs sunlight and fresh air and movement.

Like NEAT, plants improve your well-being and productivity. Texas A&M researchers found that volunteers who kept flowers and plants in their workspace were more productive than those who worked in a plant-free workplace. More remarkably, a brain scan study by Kansas State University researchers found that women's brains were significantly less stressed when they worked next to a plant than when they typed away at a bare desk. As if that weren't enough, NASA research has shown that houseplants can reduce concentrations of toxic gasses like formaldehyde, benzol, and trichloroethylene in the air, as well as provide a healthy level of humidity in the inside environment. Above all, they add vitality to a barren landscape of metal, machine, and fluorescent lights. Your plant helps keep you connected to the vast outdoors in a world that keeps us indoors far too long.

Don't have a green thumb? Look for succulents like burro's tail or aloe vera that don't mind if you forget to water them. Pick up an ivy like bird's foot that is hardy and thrives in small pots. Or go with a shoot of bamboo — it requires some attention, but it's practically indestructible!

NEAT FUEL CELLS: Two-fuel-cell breakfast

A typical American eats nearly 30 pounds of bananas a year. So, chances are good that you'll be peeling back the skin on this portable fruit for your first few morning meals. That's perfectly fine, as bananas are indeed nutritious. As you proceed through the plan, however, I encourage you to broaden your horizons and seek out berries, tropical fruits, melons, and other brightly colored fruits that deliver antioxidants and other nutrients hard to find in other foods.

WHEN DO NEAT BEATS COUNT AS NEAT FEET?

Let's say you spend an hour roaming around an art gallery as one of your NEAT Beat activities. That is an hour of NEAT Feet activity, as well, so you can use it toward your NEAT Feet quota. Anytime your NEAT Beat has you up and on your feet at a time you would normally be doing something sedentary, you can count it toward your NEAT Feet prescription. However, I still encourage you to avoid sitting for prolonged periods of time and to aim for as much NEAT Feet time as possible. Remember those NEAT cells and fat-capturing enzymes that fall asleep during inactivity? You need continuous movement to keep them ignited and doing their job.

DAY 1 CHECKLIST: Today is a 6-point day

Check off what you did and assign yourself the appropriate number of points.

NEAT Feet: Three twenty-minute walks.

____ /____ /____

____ points (3 points: 1 for each walk)

NEAT Beat: Bought a plant. ____

____ points (2 points)

NEAT Fuel Cells: Two-fuel-cell breakfast.

____

____ point (1 point)

Grand total: ____ (out of 6 points)

Day 2: Tuesday

NEAT FEET: Three twenty-minute walks

You don't need special walking shoes to embark on your NEAT journey, but the truth is that you won't get very far if your feet hurt. Now is the time to invest in stylish yet comfortable shoes that fit. Surveys reveal that 88 percent of American women wear shoes that are too small, which is likely why women have four times as many foot problems as men. Most people's feet grow a little once they hit adulthood; so get your feet measured and shop for well-constructed (no exposed seams on the inside to rub your skin raw) and well-cushioned shoes. Look for shoes with round or oval toes and wide heels to give your feet ample space and support.

NEAT BEAT: Excuse-proof your environment

I have plenty of clients who are gung ho and 100 percent committed . . . seven to eight months out of the year. Then it gets too hot or too cold and many of them disappear. Others are waylaid by the first interruption, such as the boss calling a lunch meeting when they planned on walking. For NEAT living and all of its benefits to stick, it has to be practiced consistently. That's why I insist that my patients excuse-proof their environment. They need something they can and will do to meet their daily NEAT Feet quota regardless of the weather or circumstance. A treadmill at home in front of the TV or in the office is my personal favorite, because walking is a very natural, not disruptive, activity — you can type, talk on the phone, read a book, and so on while you do it. Other options are compact exercisers such as mini steppers that fit neatly under your desk and can help you sneak in NEAT activity when you are otherwise "stuck in the box" for the day. These devices are highly effective, and I would strongly encourage you to invest in one if leaving your office or cube is difficult during the day.

In a study of nineteen men and women, we found that by using an office-place stepping device, the volunteers boosted their metabolism by about 300 calories an hour — similar to walking and other NEAT activity. Hop on it a couple hours a day and you can shed up to 44 pounds in a year. It's hard to beat that.

You can find portable steppers and mini exercise bikes (just a set of pedals that fits under your desk) at many department and sporting goods stores, as well as online at sites like Stamina Products (www.staminaproducts.com). These devices are relatively inexpensive, most cost under $100, and they are easy to use absolutely anywhere. And they work, as NEAT tester Lisa Daily of Sarasota, Florida, found while using one for a story in *Woman's World* magazine. "I used my portable cycle for two hours a day while working on my computer and sometimes while watching TV in the evening with my husband. I set the resistance pretty low so it was easy to pedal and I definitely didn't break a sweat, and I still lost five pounds the first week and four pounds the week after that — more than a size in two weeks! It was unbelievable. I had been trying exercise to lose weight forever. I even hired a trainer three times a week. The big difference was being able to do it while I was typing or talking on the phone. It was so easy, I would forget I was doing it. What also surprised me was how much more focused I was while I was working. As a writer, I spend long days in front of my computer, and it gets tiring. I often get up and take snack breaks or drink a lot of caffeine to stay alert, especially in the afternoon. When I was busy moving my body, my brain worked better! I didn't feel the need to get up and get a snack. I worked more effectively for longer stretches. And I didn't have that 3 o'clock drop; my energy was even all day long. I love it!"

NEAT FUEL CELLS: Two-fuel-cell breakfast

"But I get sick if I eat in the morning!" I've heard that lament from more than one breakfast-phobic patient, who complains that they not only don't have an appetite first thing in the morning; but that the mere sight of food flips their stomach. An a.m.

meal is essential to fuel your metabolism and avoid overeating later in the day; but it needn't be a lot of food. If you're a breakfast skipper, try just eating your fruit first thing and saving the rest of your morning meal for a little later when your stomach is settled. Or try having a small bite and then taking your morning walk. Some of my clients find that a little activity is all they need to spark their appetite.

DAY 2 CHECKLIST: Today is a 6-point day

NEAT Feet: Three twenty-minute walks.
_____ /_____ /_____
_____ points (3 points: 1 for each walk)

NEAT Beat: Excuse-proofed your
environment. _____
Write your top three excuses and
your top three solutions.

_____

_____

_____

_____ points (2 points)

NEAT Fuel Cells: Two-fuel-cell breakfast.

____

____ point (1 point)

Grand total: ____ (out of 6 points)

Day 3: Wednesday

NEAT FEET: Three twenty-minute walks

The third day of any new endeavor is an important milestone. You've been at it just long enough that the novelty is slightly dimmed, but not nearly long enough that it's ingrained. For that reason, the third day is actually one of the toughest for some of my patients. To keep yourself motivated, I recommend going back to page 132 and reviewing your goals. Remind yourself where you want to go with your NEAT life. Also, review the daily activity logs you filled out on pages 139–148. Check out which activities you planned to "move in the NEAT direction." Have you made any of your previously sedentary tasks more active? Have you held any walk-and-talk meetings? Have you traded in your happy hour for a stroll through the park with a friend? Have you taken your kids to the park today so you could all get more NEAT? If the answer is no, now is the time to push those red activities into the green and keep your forward momentum. Where will your feet take you today? Make it somewhere good.

If there is no way to leave your office for even a short walking meeting or solo brainstorm, *get up* out of your chair and stand, and, if possible, pace. This counts as NEAT activity and is the very least you can do for your health.

NEAT BEAT: Revisit your NEAT Treats

What better day to think about rewarding your "sticktoitivism" than Day 3? Stay on track and you'll be able to reward yourself at the end of next week. Review your NEAT Treats on page 202 and start thinking specifically about your rewards, if you have not done so yet. For instance, if your first reward is "a new dress," pick a specific style and write it down. Also, now that you have the hang of what the NEAT life looks like, feel free to go back and tinker with your list a little. Think broadly. Remember you don't have to *buy* yourself something. Maybe you take a full day to yourself to do whatever you wish. Or maybe you buy something small but significant, like a new cooking knife for chopping vegetables or a personal blender for whipping up breakfast smoothies. Whatever you choose, make sure it's special and preferably linked in some way to NEAT living. CDs, DVDs, and the like are nice, but most of us buy these items anyway, so they won't provide much motivation or carry any real significance.

You are rewarding your behavior — performing your NEAT Feets and NEAT Beats and following the NEAT Fuel Cell System — not your outcome. Too often, weight loss or fitness plans reward end results, such as losing 5, 15, or 30 pounds, but not the behaviors it takes to get there. So, in effect, they can end up rewarding some rather unhealthy or completely unsustainable behaviors, like starving oneself or fad dieting. In the NEAT Plan, you are rewarding yourself for changing your behaviors with rewards that will in turn help you continue those new, improved behaviors. Eventually, the behaviors themselves and the improved energy, mood, and fitness they impart will be more than enough reward.

NEAT FUEL CELLS: Two-fuel-cell breakfast

One easy way to include fruit with your breakfast is to literally make the fruit part of your breakfast via a smoothie. If you're time pressed in the mornings, don't care to sit down to a meal, and/or want a fresh alternative to your typical "breakfast bar," smoothies are a perfect solution. Here is one of my favorite one-fuel-cell recipes. You can even make a big batch and freeze it in single serving cups, so you can literally just grab it and go.

Try any variation of this recipe: 1/2 cup milk (skim or soy), 1/2 frozen banana, 1/2 cup yogurt (try lemon or another light flavor), 1 cup favorite fruit (preferably frozen, no sugar added), and a drizzle of honey to taste.

DAY 3 CHECKLIST: Today is a 6-point day

NEAT Feet: Three twenty-minute walks.
_____ / _____ / _____
_____ points (3 points: 1 for each walk)

NEAT Beat: Finalized my NEAT Treats.
_____
_____ points (2 points)

NEAT Fuel Cells: Two-fuel-cell breakfast.
_____
_____ point (1 point)

Grand total: _____ (out of 6 points)

Day 4: Thursday

NEAT FEET: Three twenty-minute walks

"Where do I put my stuff?" That's a commonly asked question clients ask as they begin integrating their NEAT walks into their work life. They're eager to take to their feet, but with just two hands and often limited pocket space, it's a juggling act to carry their notepad, pen, BlackBerry, Dictaphone, laptop, and/or other mobile office equipment they wish to bring along on their journey. Some opt to simply bring their usual briefcase or purse. That's fine if you have just a few light items; but add a laptop, and it can be a burden on your back and shoulders in just a few blocks. A better choice is a backpack (and, yes, you can get lovely leather "professional" packs that look like you're going to the office, not the Alps), which allows you to carry the weight close to your body and distributes the load evenly, so as not to overly stress either side of your body. Or, if you need quick, on-the-go access to the contents of your bag (e.g., to write notes or make calls), you can opt for a messenger bag, which has one wide strap that sits on one shoulder and crosses the chest to allow the bag to sit against the lower back and be swiveled forward on command. Just be sure the bag you use has a waist strap to keep the bag in place as you walk, so the weight stays put and doesn't bounce against you or ride around to your hip, where it will put undue strain on one side of your body.

NEAT BEAT: Fasten your NEAT Belt

When my clients start gaining weight, the first thing many do is slip into their baggy clothes. That's a mistake if you want to lose weight because too-large clothes send your brain the message that your weight is A-OK; in fact, since your clothes are so loose, your brain actually thinks you can probably afford to eat more if you like. Those large, formless clothes provide zero stimulation to your muscles and do not inspire NEAT movement. Wearing something slightly snug, on the other hand, is a reminder to your muscles (and your mind) to get up and move and to be mindful of the fuels you choose.

That's why today's NEAT Beat is a belt. Go to a drugstore and pick up a roll of elastic tape. It should be 1/2- to 1-inch thick. Snip off a strand that is about 8 inches larger than your waist. Tie it around your waist, so it is stretched and snug, but is in no way digging into your skin or cutting off circulation. Take a pen and make a mark by the knot (as you lose weight and need to tighten the belt, you will be able to see how many inches you've lost). This is your personal NEAT Belt. You can certainly take it off to sleep and shower, but you should fasten it every morning to prepare yourself for another day on the NEAT journey. It will also help cue your core muscles (the ones in your abdominal area) to stay taut to support erect, active posture and will serve as an ever-present reminder to get up and move whenever possible. Do not put off this Beat; it is essential. I have had clients lose significant amounts of weight doing little more than wearing their NEAT Belt.

NEAT FUEL CELLS: Two-fuel-cell breakfast

Add one fruit or vegetable to your lunch.

Today you begin including a fruit or vegetable at lunch, as well. Though french fries and potato chips are technically made from vegetables, they don't count here. It should be easily recognizable and as fresh as possible. Think apples, grapes, a side salad, baby carrots, grape tomatoes, cucumber or bell pepper slices, or any other colorful produce.

DAY 4 CHECKLIST: Today is a 7-point day

NEAT Feet: Three twenty-minute walks.
____ / ____ / ____
____ points (3 points: 1 for each walk)

NEAT Beat: Bought and fastened my
NEAT Belt. ____
____ points (3 points . . . *very* important;
do it now)

NEAT Fuel Cells: Two-fuel-cell breakfast
and fruit or vegetable with lunch. ____
____ point (1 point)

Grand total: ____ (out of 7 points)

Day 5: Friday

NEAT FEET: Three twenty-minute walks

Multitasking during your walks does not
have to be all business. In fact, some of my
most successful clients make their walks all
pleasure. "My wife and I lead busy lives,"
said Jeremy, a thirty-eight-year-old sales
representative who lost 10 pounds. "So the
only time we actually get to catch up with
each other without all these other demands

is when we head out for a walk." This is a perfect example of what researchers call "active intimacy" — spending quality time engaging with your partner, using both your bodies and minds, without distraction. If you've been going the NEAT journey alone, now might be a good time to enlist a friend, preferably your spouse. Stanford University researchers found that adults who start a wellness program with their partners are much more likely to stick to it and far less likely to drop out than those who go it alone. Find someone to join you for one of your walks today.

NEAT BEAT: Write tomorrow's to-dos

The weekends were made for NEAT. Even if you struggle to break the chains to your desk Monday through Friday, you likely have leisure time on the weekends to pursue all sorts of NEAT activity, from home repair to going out to a driving range to going dancing. For today's NEAT Beat, I want you to mentally explore all those possibilities and write down five things you can do to increase your NEAT on weekends (if you have ideas for the weekdays, write those down, too!). Then plan a NEAT activity for tomorrow and write it down on the checklist on the following page.

Chances are your NEAT activities will actually be things you *want* to do but just haven't made time for. If you hope to make them a reality, you must remove any obstacles that kept you from doing them. For instance, maybe in the back of your mind you have been wanting to paint the dining room, but it just falls by the wayside because it seems like an overwhelming job and you just can't get motivated to start. Like pushing a boulder down a cliff, it only takes one small step to get it in motion. So, right now, next to your NEAT activities I want you to write the one small step you need to take to get those NEAT activities under way. In the dining room example, it might take nothing more complicated than going to the hardware store and picking up paint swatches to hang on the walls. When you see the swatches, you'll be inspired to take the next step, and so on and so on. Likewise, maybe you've wanted to learn ballroom dance, but don't know where to go. Your one small step could be to pick up the Yellow Pages and write down the numbers of some dance studios that offer beginner classes for adults. One small step can get even the biggest goals in motion.

NEAT FUEL CELLS: Two-fuel-cell breakfast

Add one fruit or vegetable to your lunch.

In a head-to-head comparison of nineteen commonly eaten fruits, cranberries topped the list in antioxidant power, closely followed by blueberries and blackberries. Dried cranberries (without added sugar) are delicious in oatmeal, and blackberries and blueberries are a wonderful addition to any breakfast cereal or smoothie. Or just eat them as a snack or dessert. Remember, they're unlimited in the NEAT Plan.

DAY 5 CHECKLIST: Today is a 6-point day

NEAT Feet: Three twenty-minute walks.

____ /____ /____

____ points (3 points: 1 for each walk)

NEAT Beat: Wrote a list of five NEAT activities and planned tomorrow's NEAT activity. ____

Tomorrow I will:

My five NEAT activities and the small

steps to make them happen:

1. _____
2. _____
3. _____
4. _____
5. _____

_____ points (2 points)

_____

_____

NEAT Fuel Cells: Two-fuel-cell breakfast and one fruit or vegetable with lunch.

_____

_____ point (1 point)

_____

_____

Grand total: _____ (out of 6 points)

_____

Day 6: Saturday

NEAT FEET: Three twenty-minute walks

Not sure where your feet are going to take you this weekend? Try this: Go to Google Maps and find a street map of the nearest town where you go shopping, visit the library, buy groceries, and so on. Take a pen and mark all the places you know or frequently go, including stores, parks, the post office, and friends' houses. Now, take a highlighter and start connecting these destinations. Using the map scale, indicate the distance between each point. Figure that it will take you about twenty minutes to walk (purposefully) 1 mile or thirty minutes to stroll the distance. You're likely surprised to see how many of your favorite places are within a 1-mile radius of one another. Post this map on your refrigerator or bulletin board and use it as a reference when you're looking for more places you can travel via foot. Next time you're going into town, just park in a central location and walk the rest.

NEAT BEAT: Get camera ready

First, be sure to do the NEAT activity you planned for today. Then, for today's NEAT Beat, find your camera and make sure the battery is charged and it's ready to roll. Next, find out what time sunrise is in your area tomorrow. (Weather.com, the newspaper, or any weather station will give you this information.) Set your alarm for this time. Just a heads-up (since chances are you don't read this book before sunrise), because tomorrow's NEAT Beat will be photographing the sunrise. So find a good spot in your house or yard where you can get a good shot!

Yes, it'll be early, but that's the point. NEAT living is about embracing each day to its fullest and finding time to live a full, active life. Maybe you won't always get up at the crack of dawn on a Sunday morning, but by doing so tomorrow, you'll have the opportunity to experience how wide open and full of possibilities and potential each day really is, especially when you're on the go before most of the rest of the world has roused.

NEAT FUEL CELLS: Two-fuel-cell breakfast

Add one fruit or vegetable to your lunch.

I know people who don't buy fresh produce because they claim they don't eat it fast enough and fear that most of the nutrients are leeched out by the time they do. That shouldn't be a problem on the NEAT Plan, since fresh produce is unlimited and mandatory with meals. But it's also not an excuse, because it's not true, at least as far as the produce's antioxidants are concerned. A recent study by Belgian researchers found that storage, either in the fridge or at room temperature, did not result in the loss of any of the essential antioxidants, including phenols, flavonols, or ascorbic acid. In some cases, the antioxidant capacity actually *increased* as the produce further ripened. So long as you eat it before it spoils, your produce will still provide valuable health protection.

DAY 6 CHECKLIST: Today is a 7-point day

NEAT Feet: Three 20-minute walks.
_____ /_____ /_____
_____ points (3 points: 1 for each walk)

NEAT Beat: Camera is ready; alarm is set. _____
_____ points (3 points)

NEAT Fuel Cells: Two-fuel-cell breakfast and one fruit or vegetable with lunch. _____
_____ point (1 point)

Grand total: _____ (out of 7 points)

Saturday is weigh-in day: Weigh yourself in the morning and jot the number here. _____

Day 7: Sunday

NEAT FEET: Three twenty-minute walks

The human machine is built to walk. But if you've taken more steps during these past six days than you've taken over the past six years, there's a chance you're feeling a little sore, especially if you've been walking at a pace that is brisker than typical human locomotion (e.g., faster than about 1 to 2 miles per hour). I don't want to discourage you from picking up your pace, of course; but I also don't want you to get sidelined by soreness. The easiest way to keep aches and pains at bay is to stay loose by stretching when you're done.

One walkers' stretch I love is the heel drop. Stand on the edge of a step with the balls of your feet on the step. Now drop your heels so you feel a stretch in your feet, Achilles tendon region, and calves. Hold for twenty to thirty seconds. You can also do one foot at a time for a deeper stretch.

When you're done, stretch your hamstrings by propping your flexed right heel on the step with the right leg extended and bending the left knee slightly as you lean forward from the hips. Hold twenty to thirty seconds; then switch legs.

NEAT BEAT: Photograph the sunrise

Have you ever had a terrible night where you had an argument with a loved one, a child came home way past curfew and scared you to pieces, or you laid awake late into the night overwhelmed with anxiety only to arise the next day to see the sun shining and feel the comforting relief of a new day wash over you? That is the power of the sunrise. It symbolizes a new beginning. It is filled with promise. It renews and regenerates us.

The same can be said of NEAT. As you've likely noticed by now, this is not just any fitness book. NEAT transcends the realm of physical fitness and reaches into the very essence of life itself — movement. Every single time you move, you make something happen. Every NEAT action, whether it's something as simple as combing your hair a new way today or calling an old friend to go bird watching, has a ripple effect that changes your life. Every step on the NEAT journey can take you somewhere you've never been but always wanted to go. By the end of these eight weeks, I don't want for you to have just lost weight. I want that weight loss to be a by-product of living your life in a whole new way — an unnecessary burden you left behind in the darkness of yesterday as you stepped into the dawning light of a new day.

NEAT FUEL CELLS: Two-fuel-cell breakfast
Add one fruit or vegetable to your lunch.

Even if you eat lunch out every day, getting your mandatory fruit or vegetable should be no problem at all. In fact, you should be able to get two or more easily. Start with your sandwich. Lettuce, tomatoes, sprouts, spinach, shaved carrots, roasted peppers, sliced mushrooms, and all the other assorted toppings you'll find at many delis are delicious, easy ways to fuel up on vegetables. Add a piece of fruit and it's a complete dish.

DAY 7 CHECKLIST: Today is a 7-point day

NEAT Feet: Three twenty-minute walks.

_____ / _____ / _____

_____ points (3 points: 1 for each walk)

NEAT Beat: Photographed the sunrise.

_____

Print out your photo (or draw a picture of it as a placeholder in the meantime) here. It is the dawn of your new NEAT life.

_____ points (2 points)

Dawn

NEAT Fuel Cells: Two-fuel-cell breakfast and one fruit or vegetable with lunch. ____
____ point (1 point)

Grand total: ____ (out of 7 points)

END-OF-WEEK ADD-UP

Maximum points: 45
My points: _____

8
WEEK 2: DREAM IT, DO IT

Welcome to Week 2, a seven-day stretch of big thoughts and NEAT actions. This week, I'm going to ask you to flip back and review your NEAT Goal Sheet (see page 132). Your NEAT Beats will focus around these goals, as well as the NEAT activities you planned last week. Ideally, these two facets of your life will begin to dovetail as your NEAT activities bring you closer to your goals. But it's okay if that's not the case right out of the gate. By participating in any NEAT activity, you are forging the habit of living an active, highly engaged life — a crucial first step to realizing any big dream. Speaking of active, your NEAT Feet prescription steps it up a notch this week, as one walk per day gets longer. And you'll be following the NEAT Fuel Cell System for both breakfast and lunch all week for your NEAT Fuel Cells, as well as incorporating the other NEAT fueling tenets. You are now firmly on the path to a new you!

Day 1: Monday

NEAT FEET: Two twenty-minute walks; one thirty-minute walk

For decades, thirty minutes has been the official benchmark for minimum daily exercise. The Aerobics and Fitness Association of America recently reported that if you walk briskly for thirty minutes each day, you'll shed between 16 to 18 pounds a year without doing anything else. Starting this week, you'll be meeting that thirty-minute mark with just one of your NEAT Feet walks. You'll note that I don't generally recommend any particular pace for walking. NEAT is a journey, not a destination. Your walks should be enjoyable, not punishing or painful. That's why I rarely recommend walking faster for the sake of walking faster. The most important, and effective, strategy is to simply get in the habit of being up and on your feet, not rushing down the road.

NEAT BEAT: Do one of the five NEAT activities you planned on page 230

The secret to successful NEAT activities is simplicity. When I ask patients to draw up a list of activities, inevitably some will go overboard with their ambition. Like Jane, a mother of two in her early forties, whose list looked like this:

1. Clean all my closets.
2. Clear out the basement.
3. Organize the attic.

And so on. These are certainly NEAT activities. But there are two problems. One, they're too ambiguous. What exactly did she mean by "clear out the basement"? In truth, she wasn't even sure (hence, when she got down there, she wasn't sure where to start and ended up quitting after five minutes). Two, they're too big. Maybe after successfully cleaning one closet, Jane would be motivated to tackle more. But cleaning *all* of them? Discouraged from the start, Jane didn't get very far. A smarter strategy is to start small and build on your success. Like Jim, a human resources manager in his late thirties, who started *really* small, and has lost 11 pounds in the process. "My three-year-old daughter likes me to hang around until she falls asleep because she's scared of the dark. I used to just lie on the floor, which nearly put me to sleep, too. So I made it a goal to use that time for activity. I started telling her I was patrolling right outside her room, and I'd walk up and down the hall, circling around through the dining room. Once she fell asleep, I'd keep up the momentum for other household activities."

NEAT FUEL CELLS: Two-fuel-cell breakfast; two-fuel-cell lunch

Despite what 1980s-era government officials may tell you, ketchup is not considered a vegetable. It's entirely too processed and sugary to qualify. But freshly made salsa (note that I said freshly made; that means in your kitchen, not from a jar) can certainly contribute to your fresh produce intake. Salsa is easy to make by mixing chopped tomatoes, onions, chili peppers, and cilantro, and goes with everything from sandwiches to sliced, toasted tortillas.

DAY 1 CHECKLIST: Today is a 6-point day

NEAT Feet: Two twenty-minute walks; one thirty-minute walk. ____ /____

____ points (2 points: 1 for *both* twenty-minute walks; 1 for the thirty-minute walk)

NEAT Beat: Did one of my five planned

NEAT activities. _____
_____ points (2 points)

NEAT Fuel Cells: Two-fuel-cell breakfast.
_____
Two-fuel-cell lunch. _____
_____ points (2 points: 1 for each meal)

Grand total: _____ (out of 6 points)

Day 2: Tuesday

NEAT FEET: Two twenty-minute walks; one thirty-minute walk

When my clients complain of pains from ramping up their walking schedule, they're usually from the knees down. That's because those muscles and connective tissues that would be naturally strong from standing and walking have weakened from years of relative inactivity. Generally, the more you walk, the stronger you'll get. But if you've been sedentary for a long time and are carrying some extra weight, you may need to strengthen your muscles to support your joints and keep aches and pains at bay. Here are two moves I recommend. They can easily be done in the morning or evening and will take less than two minutes.

Straight Knee Leg Lifts: Sit on the floor with legs extended straight in front of you. Bend one knee and place that foot on the floor, while keeping the other leg straight. Contract the thigh muscle of the straight leg, so you feel the kneecap engage. Now lift the extended leg several inches off the ground and hold for about five seconds. Lower the leg back down to the floor. Relax for a second. Repeat five more times. Then switch legs.

Toe Taps: Sit on the floor with legs extended straight in front of you. Flex your feet and draw your toes straight back toward your knees. Hold for about five seconds. Now point your toes away from you, pushing the soles of your feet toward the floor. Hold for about five seconds. Repeat each move five more times.

NEAT BEAT: Do one of the five NEAT activities you planned on page 230, but not the same one as yesterday

Compare today's NEAT activity to yesterday's. Are they similar or completely different? You're likely eager to infuse NEAT into every aspect of your life, which, of course, is the ultimate goal. But in the beginning, you may find more satisfaction (and thereby success) by linking your NEAT activities together to achieve one specific goal. For instance, if you have been longing to do some minor remodeling in your kitchen, it makes perfect sense to focus your NEAT activities on that particular home improvement. One day's activity may be removing old wallpaper from around the stove. The next day's activity may be removing the wallpaper from around the refrigerator. The third day, you would move to another area of the kitchen, until the wallpaper was done. Then plot your NEAT activities around the next phase of the remodeling. Using NEAT activity this way is tremendously satisfying, because in the end you are rewarded with concrete results from your efforts. If you'll remember, this is also the essence of NEAT: using activity to achieve work (and play) in life.

NEAT FUEL CELLS: Two-fuel-cell breakfast; two-fuel-cell lunch

What do oatmeal and soup have in common? They're quick meals that are begging to be embellished with lots of fresh fruits and/or vegetables. By folding in fistfuls of blueberries, diced apple, pear chunks, raspberries, blackberries, even cherries, you take oatmeal from a ho-hum start to the day to a morning meal brimming with flavor and fiber. Likewise, by adding vegetables such as roasted red peppers and corn to store-bought soup, you amplify your enjoyment of the meal and its nutritional value. You don't need to give up those easy meals; just improve them.

Note: Tomorrow starts Slow-Food Wednesday (no fast food), so be prepared!

DAY 2 CHECKLIST: Today is a 6-point day

NEAT Feet: Two twenty-minute walks; one thirty-minute walk. ____ /____ ____ points (2 points: 1 for *both* twenty-minute walks; 1 for the thirty-minute walk)

NEAT Beat: Did another one of my five planned NEAT activities. ____

Now that you're getting the hang of NEAT activities, make some notes about how you can focus your activities to achieve long-standing goals and desires, such as having an organized garage or a cheerfully decorated kitchen.

_____
_____
_____
_____

_____ points (2 points)

NEAT Fuel Cells: Two-fuel-cell
breakfast. _____
Two-fuel-cell lunch _____.
_____ points (2 points: 1 for each meal)

Grand total: _____ (out of 6 points)

Day 3: Wednesday

NEAT FEET: Two twenty-minute walks; one thirty-minute walk

At this point, you should be using your feet to take you lots of places throughout the day. As mentioned last week, you don't need special shoes, just comfortable ones for the majority of your NEAT endeavors. Some of my patients find that they do want to walk more quickly than their everyday shoes will comfortably allow. If you find that to be a problem as you expand your NEAT walking, by all means invest in a pair of walking shoes. But be sure they are walking, not running, shoes. Running shoes tend to be built up in the heel to provide shock absorption and are stiff to control the motion of the foot during that activity. But walking uses your leg muscles much differently than running,

246

and those same stiff, shockproof shoes that will keep you comfortable on the run can actually cause sore shins and fatigue when you walk in them. Walking shoes have a more flexible sole with more bend in the toe to allow you to take natural heel-toe strides in comfort. They do not have to be expensive. Comfort is key.

NEAT BEAT: Plan a NEAT activity for Thursday

Review your notes regarding your NEAT activities from the past two days. Now go ahead and plan a NEAT activity for tomorrow from your earlier list. You can link it to the NEAT activities you've already done to build momentum. Or you can take a fresh step forward in a new direction to start working toward another larger goal. Remember, too, that the NEAT activities you choose during the week should be somewhat different than those you choose for the weekend. You may find that you long for more fun activities during the week, when so much of your time is filled with work and family obligations. If that is the case, by all means plan something lighthearted and enjoyable. Try your hand at watercolor painting. Go bowling. Play Frisbee in the backyard with your kids. Remember, NEAT is play as well as work. And it doesn't have to take all day.

Even a five-minute activity counts.

NEAT FUEL CELLS: Two-fuel-cell breakfast; two-fuel-cell lunch; No-Fast-Food Wednesday

If you haven't already been observing Slow-Food Wednesday, start today! Of course, no fast food doesn't mean that you can't eat quick meals. You just have to make them or seek them out yourself, away from the drive-through windows of McQuickie Burger. You may still go to your favorite deli, where fresh, low-fat, nonfried food can be put together in less than five minutes. You may also go to the supermarket or corner grocery, where you'll find yogurt, fruit, baby carrots, and other "fast-meal" fixings. After one or two weeks of training your taste buds away from the overly processed and salt-saturated meals served up in most fast-food joints, you may find that you prefer every day to be no-fast-food day.

DAY 3 CHECKLIST: Today is a 6-point day

NEAT Feet: Two twenty-minute walks; one thirty-minute walk. ____ /____ ____ points (2 points: 1 for *both* twenty-minute walks; 1 for the thirty-minute walk)

NEAT Beat: Planned a NEAT activity for Thursday. ____
Make a few notes about your NEAT activity for tomorrow, including what it is and when you will do it.

_____

_____

_____

_____

____ points (2 points)

NEAT Fuel Cells: Two-fuel-cell breakfast / two-fuel-cell lunch. ____
Slow-Food Wednesday. ____
____ points (2 points: 1 for *both* meals; 1 for avoiding fast food)

Grand total: ____ (out of 6 points)

Day 4: Thursday

NEAT FEET: Two twenty-minute walks; one thirty-minute walk

Walking, and sometimes even dancing, on cobblestone paths is an ancient healing activity rooted in traditional Chinese medicine. Practitioners believe that the uneven surface of the cobblestones stimulate acupressure points on the feet that promote improved organ function and health. Men and women in China often spend thirty minutes each day walking on beautiful stone paths throughout their towns and cities, and it turns out (not surprisingly) that this traditional activity is scientifically sound. In a sixteen-week study of 108 men and women over the age of sixty, scientists at the Oregon Research Institute found that those who walked on special mats made to simulate cobblestones for one-hour periods three days per week lowered their blood pressure and had better scores on measures of balance and physical function than those who spent the same amount of time walking on regular walking paths. Of course, cobblestones aren't terribly common in the United States, so you may not be able to find a quaint stone path for your daily jaunts. But you can seek out a variety of surfaces to enrich your walking experience and maybe boost your benefits. Soft surfaces such as grass, sand, and wood chip paths, for instance, force your muscles to work harder to propel you forward, since your feet sink a bit with every foot strike. This alone is an excellent way to strengthen your legs and burn more calories.

NEAT BEAT: Write about your perfect vacation, either one you've already taken or one you would like to take

What about this trip appeals to you? For most of us, vacations are a much-needed opportunity to recharge our batteries. We long for a few days with nothing to do but lie on a beach. Not surprising, after one day of nothing, most people find themselves wanting to do *something*. So they fill the time with eating, drinking, and shopping, which would be okay, except such activities often lead to feelings of guilt or remorse and very often weight gain, which leads to more of the above.

If that sounds familiar, it may be time to consider planning a NEAT vacation this year. NEAT or "active" vacations are trips built around a physical activity such as cycling, trekking, kayaking, or hiking. They can be as exotic as jungle exploration in South America or as simple as canoeing a local river. The point is to stimulate your mind and body in a fresh, new way, which you'll likely find is more regenerating than doing nothing, because you're so occupied exploring and learning and experiencing that you don't have time to even think of work, let alone check your e-mail or call into the office. The best part is that you don't have to be an experienced horseback rider or cyclist to participate. Most tour operators run beginner-friendly trips, which gives you the opportunity to try something new in a safe, fun, supportive environment. Many companies also offer family trips, so you can take the kids (or grandkids). A client of mine recently booked her dream cycling vacation to the Grand Canyon. In the mornings, she and her husband did long bike rides with the adults, while the kids enjoyed planned, supervised activities, such as fossil hunts. After lunch, the tour operator offered easier family rides that were open to children as young as six.

As part of today's NEAT Beat, Google "active vacations" and peruse the incredible array of active opportunities available for your next trip. Here is just a sampling of what you will find.

Adventure cruises
Archaeological tours
ATV tours
Backcountry skiing
Bicycle and mountain biking tours
Canoeing
Cattle drives
City tours

Cross-country skiing
Culinary vacations
Cultural tours
Dog sledding
Drama camp
Dude and guest ranches
Ecotourism and jungle exploration
Fishing charters
Golf vacations
Hiking and trekking tours
Horse pack trips and trail rides
Kayaking
Mountain and rock climbing
Multisport adventures
Safaris
Sailing vacations
Scuba diving
Surfing camps
Swimming with dolphins
Wagon train trips
Walking tours
Whale-watching tours
White-water rafting
Wildlife-viewing tours
Yoga retreats

After reading, has your idea of an ideal vacation changed?

NEAT FUEL CELLS: Two-fuel-cell breakfast; two-fuel-cell lunch

There's a saying in business: Fail to plan, plan to fail. Some are naturally more inclined to plan, while others fly a bit more by the seat of our pants. The latter doesn't work so well when it comes to following healthy eating habits, especially since our society is a minefield of overprocessed saturated fat and sugar bombs at every turn. It's easier to navigate this calorie-littered landscape when you are armed with healthful foods whenever you need them. That means stocking more than your home pantry and refrigerator. It means stashing fruit and nuts in your office or in your purse or briefcase if you work outside the home, and in your car if you're frequently on the go. That way you can stick to your fuel cell plan wherever you are.

DAY 4 CHECKLIST: Today is a 7-point day

NEAT Feet: Two twenty-minute walks; one thirty-minute walk. ____ /____ ____ points (2 points: 1 for *both* twenty-minute walks; 1 for the thirty-minute walk)

NEAT Beat: Write about your perfect

vacation, either one you've already taken or one you would like to take.
Make a few notes about what kind of NEAT vacation you may enjoy.

_____

_____

_____

_____

_____

_____ points (3 points; put some effort into this and narrow it down to two or three real possibilities. Start planning!)

_____

_____

NEAT Fuel Cells: Two-fuel-cell breakfast. _____
Two-fuel-cell lunch. _____
_____ points (2 points: 1 for each meal)

_____

_____

Grand total: _____ (out of 7 points)

_____

Day 5: Friday

NEAT FEET: Two twenty-minute walks; one thirty-minute walk

Remember, though walking is an ideal NEAT activity, it's not the only one that counts toward your NEAT Feet goals. Skating, gardening, yoga, Pilates, perusing an art gallery, or anything that keeps you on your feet moving for at least thirty minutes counts.

NEAT BEAT: Answer this question: What do you want from life?

There's a big one, huh? You started to explore this on your NEAT Goal Sheet. But those dreams are just part of your NEAT life. Now it's time to dig deeper and explore what your life would look like in an ideal world. In your utterly, totally, amazing dream life, what would you be doing? What are the things that would make it so amazing? Happiness? Success? Monetary comfort? How close are you to your dream life? What is standing in your way? You may be surprised to learn that it's a lack of NEAT. Remember, NEAT is the energy of life. It is motion taking you somewhere and accomplishing something. The sedentary inertia that has overtaken modern life is the enemy of NEAT and the biggest barrier standing between you and your dreams.

Take for example Renee, a forty-seven-year-old office manager. She was 60 pounds overweight and stuck in a dead-end job. Her husband had had an affair and left her three years prior, and she was miserable. At the time, she thought her weight was her biggest problem. But her weight, though it did literally weigh her down, was simply a symptom of the larger concern — lack of movement. She was stuck and needed just one good shove to get her rolling in the right direction. Instead of offering up a weight-loss program or a dietary plan, I quizzed her about her social life, hoping to tap into some of her anger. As it bubbled to the surface, I saw how much potential energy she had bottled up! I encouraged her to harness her fury to change her life. The first thing she did was start hunting for new jobs. A year later, she had a new job and a new man and was 40 pounds lighter without ever actually dieting or "exercising." All she did was move toward her dream life and her weight melted away.

Now it's your turn. What "push" do you need? If you can't get the job of your dreams without a degree, start investigating classes. If your marriage is stale, plan a NEAT vacation with your spouse to infuse it with excitement. Staying where you are may feel safe and comfortable, but if it's not making you happy, you must push out of that comfort zone. Being successful takes effort, sometimes a lot of effort. But the journey is invigorating, and every step takes you closer to your dreams.

NEAT FUEL CELLS: Two-fuel-cell breakfast; two-fuel-cell lunch; Fat-free Friday

If you haven't already, now is the time to introduce Fat-free Fridays into your meal plan. Remember, this does not include healthy fats naturally found in almonds or salmon. These are foods made with fat or have fat added, such as cookies, cakes, potato chips, creams, candy bars, fried foods, and heavy sauces or dips such as cheese dip and Alfredo sauce. Your goal is to eat food that is as clean and light as possible. Make note of how much lighter and energetic you feel when you eat like this, especially if it is a drastic departure from your usual Friday fare.

DAY 5 CHECKLIST: Today is a 7-Point Day

NEAT Feet: Two twenty-minute walks; one thirty-minute walk. ____ /____ ____ points (2 points: 1 for *both* twenty-minute walks; 1 for the thirty-minute walk)

NEAT Beat: Answer this question: What do you want from life? Write it down now.

_____ points (3 points; this is essential.)

NEAT Fuel Cells: Two-fuel-cell breakfast; two-fuel-cell lunch. _____
Fat-free Friday. _____
_____ points (2 points: 1 for both meals; 1 for going fat free)

Grand total: _____ (out of 7 points)

Day 6: Saturday

NEAT FEET: Two twenty-minute walks; one thirty-minute walk

One of the tenets of the NEAT journey is to be generous. Make it a goal to use one of your walks today for an act of generosity. This can be as simple as walking over to say hi to a neighbor you haven't seen in a while, or it can be stopping by a florist and picking up a bouquet of flowers for a friend who's been going through a rough spell. It can be gathering all those old clothes you've been meaning to donate and taking them to the drop-off bin. Think of an act of kindness you can do today and do it.

NEAT BEAT: Begin planning to make your dream life a reality

Bring a pad and paper on one of today's walks and write down the ten steps you need to take to make your dream life a reality. This list should include small as well as big steps. Take at least one small step today.

A perfect example is Jane, a single mother of two young children who was struggling to make ends meet working at a fast-food restaurant. She was about 50 pounds overweight, depressed, and scared of the future. In her dream life, she was healthy and happy and had a fulfilling job that allowed her to work regular hours and support her family without scraping by. On the surface, her dream life seemed unattainable. But she was smart. She started with one very small step: researching the state resources available to single moms. With just a little digging, she found a program that provided day care and other accommodations while mothers earned a college degree. The next big step was to attend one lecture. "I still remember the first day I went to that college," recalled Jane. "I was nearly too scared to go, but my mom said I had to attend just one lecture, and then I could quit if I really wanted to. That first lecture was about how to organize a paper, and I had to write about the subject of my choice. I wrote about my kids' first day of day care. I got an A." The rest, as they say, is history, including her weight. By taking that first step, Jane reinvented herself and her life. In three years, she became a legal assistant and lost more than 45 pounds along the way. She had incredible dreams and achieved more than she dreamed of. More important, she transformed the lives of her children, who witnessed their mother taking control of her own destiny.

Choosing what you would like to do and taking the first step toward it is where NEAT living begins. This is your one and only life. Only you can take the necessary steps to live it to its fullest. Never underestimate the power and importance of recognizing those first steps you need to take . . . and of actually taking them. It starts with planning. Once you plan, you begin to do.

NEAT FUEL CELLS: Two-fuel-cell breakfast; two-fuel-cell lunch; no eating in the car

As a rule, I preach "Don't sit when you can stand; don't stand when you can move." The one exception is eating. Eating, even snacking, should be a purposeful, mindful activity, which is a far cry from how most food is consumed in our culture today. Put every meal and snack on a plate, pull up a seat, and sit down and focus on the task at hand — savoring every bite. You'll eat less, enjoy your food more, and feel less hungry, because you've given your body a chance to register that you have fueled up. In keeping with that spirit, if you haven't already, make it a point to stop eating in the car today. We eat far too much, often out of boredom, and usually nutritionally barren food when we eat in our vehicles.

DAY 6 CHECKLIST: Today is a 7-point day

NEAT Feet: Two twenty-minute walks; one thirty-minute walk. _____ / _____ _____ points (2 points: 1 for *both* twenty-minute walks; 1 for the thirty-minute walk)

NEAT Beat: Write down the ten steps you need to take to make your dream life a reality. This list should include small as well as big steps, and should be progressive. Take at least one small step today.

1. _____
2. _____
3. _____
4. _____

5. _____

6. _____

7. _____

8. _____

9. _____

10. _____

_____ points (3 points)

NEAT Fuel Cells: Two-fuel-cell breakfast. _____

Two-fuel-cell lunch. _____

_____ points (2 points: 1 for each meal)

Grand total: _____ (out of 7 points)

Saturday is weigh-in day: Weigh yourself in the morning and jot the number here. _____

Day 7: Sunday

NEAT FEET: Two twenty-minute walks; one thirty-minute walk

Another tenet of the NEAT journey is worship. Many religions actually incorporate walking into their prayer and reflection. Others include great pilgrimages as part of their sacred rituals. It's not surprising.

Walking allows you to perform a type of moving meditation that centers the body and calms the mind. The quiet of a Sunday morning is the perfect time to practice walking meditation. Simply start walking. Focus on your breathing. Feel the air enter your lungs and energize your body as you inhale. Feel it flow out from your body and relieve your stress as you exhale. Feel your footsteps on the earth. Feel yourself becoming part of the natural world around you, breathing the air, absorbing the sun's rays, stepping on the solid ground. Your breathing will slow down as your movements become more fluid and free flowing. Notice how calm you feel, how at one with the universe you've become. Remember, you can return to this state nearly each and every time you walk.

NEAT BEAT: Make a record of your home-cooked meals

Write down how many meals you cooked at home this week (even if you took them to work and ate them there). Then look up a two-fuel-cell (400-calorie) recipe and copy it down.

Though there are literally thousands of meals that can be cooked for breakfast, lunch, or dinners, most people settle on about four. You know the drill, if it's Tuesday, it's meat loaf; Friday is pizza; and so on. It's easy to get in a food rut, which opens the door to boredom and eventually eating out because it's more interesting. The first step to avoiding this trap is simply making variations of your favorite standby meals. Always make beef tacos? Try chicken this week. Is it chicken and rice night? Go with couscous instead. Try cooking a familiar food in a different way. Roast your vegetables instead of steaming them. Stir-fry your fish. Toss it all into a Crock-Pot and make a stew. Or simply Google your favorite dish. You're guaranteed to find some recipes with interesting twists. Each time you try something even a little new, it introduces a new food, flavor, or fresh way of cooking that will spill into the next meal.

NEAT FUEL CELLS: Two-fuel-cell breakfast; two-fuel-cell lunch

While we're talking about food, yet another tenet of the NEAT journey is to share. There may be no more generous or loving act than to share a meal you've made with your own hands. As you're cooking today, make a little extra and share it with a friend, coworker, or neighbor. If you can't actually have them over to break bread, dish some into a Tupperware container and walk it over to them or bring it into work. You just might inspire someone to join you on your journey.

DAY 7 CHECKLIST: Today is a 6-point day

NEAT Feet: Two twenty-minute walks; one thirty-minute walk. ____ /____ ____ points (2 points: 1 for *both* twenty-minute walks; 1 for the thirty-minute walk)

NEAT Beat: Jot down how many meals you cooked at home this week. Copy the two-fuel-cell (400-calorie) recipe you looked up here. Also make a note of what day you'll make this new meal.

_____

____ points (2 points)

266

NEAT Fuel Cells: Two-fuel-cell breakfast.
_____

Two-fuel-cell lunch. _____
_____ (2 points: 1 for each meal)

Grand total: _____ (out of 6 points)

END-OF-WEEK ADD-UP

Maximum points: 45
My points: _____

You are a quarter of the way through the NEAT Plan. Add up your NEAT points. If you've stayed on track and hit 68 out of the possible 90, reward yourself accordingly! If not, refocus your efforts, step up to the plate, and make a change starting today.

9
Week 3: Create and Explore

NEAT is the engine that powers human exploration, invention, and progress. It is the unquenchable curiosity that compelled us to leave Africa and walk across the earth to populate it. From forging spearheads from rocks to building rocket ships to the moon, human beings have always had and continue to have the need to build and discover. Last week, we dedicated time and energy to exploring how we want our life to play out from here on into the future. We've established:

- Daily awareness of avoiding prolonged sitting and being active, rather than just thinking about it
- Planning NEAT activities, especially for the weekends
- The NEAT elastic belt reminder (time to tighten it?)
- Two-fuel-cell breakfasts and lunches
- Following NEAT eating tenets, particu-

larly Slow-Food Wednesday, Fat-free Friday, and no eating in the car

This week we will continue to infuse NEAT into your life through extended NEAT Feet activity, as well as some simple stretches and exercises to support your increase in activity. (Don't worry. These are not your typical "gym" exercises.) At this point, you should notice that your mind is brimming with ideas, solutions, and creative thought during your walks. This week's NEAT Beats will encourage you to pour some of that energy into creation and exploration. You'll now be following the fuel cell system for all three meals and becoming more of an active participant in your NEAT fueling. It's an exciting week that will let you stretch your imagination along with your legs. Let's go!

WEEKS 3 AND 4: MAKING ME A PRIORITY

I am ready to commit two hours per day to my NEAT Plan. These two weeks are about establishing:

- NEAT activity planning (create the plan; confirm the details; execute it)

- NEAT Feet activities three times a day
- Three two-fuel-cell meals per day

Along the way, I will continue to explore my goals for the future, immediate and distant, and to take steps toward expanding my NEAT life and reaching those goals. It's not always easy. But this is the only life I have, and it is happening right now. I am worth the effort, and I will make the effort.

I am ready for the next level: _____

Day 1: Monday

NEAT FEET: One twenty-minute walk; two thirty-minute walks; ten Core Chargers and five Sunrise Stretches shortly after waking

Walking is primarily a leg-based activity. But there's an important cast of characters that helps you move down the road pain-free and with impeccable posture. The muscles in your "core" — that's your abdominals, obliques (side muscles), back, and hips —

provide protective support during all NEAT activity, especially walking. When they're strong, you can hold yourself upright with ease; your back doesn't ache, and you're slower to fatigue, especially if you're also carrying a pack or shopping bags.

As you increase your NEAT Feet activity, it's important to keep these muscles up to speed. Starting each day with this core-charging exercise will do the trick.

Core Charger: Stand with your feet a few inches apart. Bend your arms and hold them out to the sides, so they form right angles with your hands toward the ceiling, palms facing forward. Contract your abs and pull your right knee and left elbow toward each other. Pause, and return to start. Then switch sides. Perform ten, five on each side.

It's equally important to keep those legs limber as you ramp up your NEAT. Your hamstrings (back of your legs) and bum put in a good day's work when you're on your feet getting lots of NEAT. It's not uncommon for them to feel a little tight now and then. Keeping them limber will help prevent discomfort. Perform these Sunrise Stretches after your Core Chargers, and you'll be good to go.

Sunrise Stretch: Stand tall. Reach your hands up toward the sky, taking a full breath and extending your body as long as possible. Exhale and sweep your arms out to the sides and body down toward the floor, reaching for your toes with your fingers. Allow your upper body to relax and be heavy, so you feel a stretch down the back of your legs. Slowly roll up to a stand, stacking one vertebra at a time as you return to the starting position. Repeat.

NEAT BEAT: Check in with yourself

You've had to do a lot these past few weeks, not the least of which was to change your lifestyle! With all these balls in the air, it can be easy to let one fall to the floor without even noticing. So take the time today to do a check-in.

- **How's your plant?** Is it thriving? Is it dead (be honest)? This living organism is symbolic of your NEAT journey. It takes attention. It takes thought. And (especially if you find it dead or dying) it takes a little knowledge. If it's not faring well, take a moment to do a little research to find out why and what it needs. If it's beyond hope, please replace it and try again, maybe with another variety, and be sure to find out how to care for it, just like you're discovering how to care for yourself.

- **Are you still wearing your NEAT Belt?** If you have trouble remembering, let your Core Chargers be your cue. Slip it on before you start your morning moves; then leave it on as a reminder to keep your core tight and stay on the NEAT path. Adjust your belt as needed as you lose weight.
- **Have you "NEAT activated" your sedentary activities?** At this point, you should have NEAT activated nearly all your sedentary activities. If you have not, make a point to activate at least one more today or tomorrow.

NEAT FUEL CELLS: Two-fuel-cell breakfast; two-fuel-cell lunch; two-fuel-cell dinner

This week, try to eat two-fuel-cell dinners. It may be hard at first, because most of us are accustomed to eating more food at dinner. If you find it too difficult, reconfigure your eating (review the examples on pages 181–186, if needed). You may need to add a fuel cell to dinner, and move one of your snacks around to keep from being hungry at another part of the day. Try it out this week, and adjust as you need to. Also keep in mind that fruits and vegetables are free. So satisfaction may be as simple as adding an apple to the end of the meal or eating a pear as you're packing your belongings to leave work at the end of the day.

DAY 1 CHECKLIST: Today is a 7-point day

NEAT Feet: One twenty-minute walk; two thirty-minute walks. _____/_____

NEAT Exercises: Ten Core Chargers and five Sunrise Stretches. _____
_____ points (3 points: 1 for *each* thirty-minute walk;
1 for the twenty-minute walk plus the NEAT exercises)

NEAT Beat: NEAT plan check-in
My plant is _____ inches tall.
I am still wearing my NEAT Belt.
Yes _____ No _____
I have NEAT activated the following sedentary activities:

I will NEAT activate the following sedentary activities:

_____

_____

_____

_____ points (2 points)

_____

_____

NEAT Fuel Cells: Two-fuel-cell breakfast.
_____

Two-fuel-cell lunch. _____
Two-fuel-cell dinner. _____
_____ points (2 points: 1 for breakfast and lunch; 1 for dinner)

_____

_____

Grand total: _____ (out of 7 points)

_____

Day 2: Tuesday

NEAT FEET: One twenty-minute walk; two thirty-minute walks; ten Core Chargers and five Sunrise Stretches shortly after waking

When a colleague of mine was designing her office, she made NEAT her primary inspiration and hired an architectural firm that created an open floor plan that encouraged getting up and milling about. You may not be able to hire a dynamic team of architectural designers to come and make over your house or workplace, but you can take a few pages from their playbook and create motion in your own space. "You want visual energy, inspiration, and plenty of reminders to get up and move," said Rachelle from Studio 2030 in Minneapolis, which specializes in creative spaces.

How can you do that? "Simple mobiles can do the trick," she said. Hang lightweight sun catchers, mobiles, or other decorations from the ceiling. They'll spin and swirl with the slightest breeze creating movement in your space. For cubicles, try dynamic decorations like mini lava lamps, sandscape desk toys, or even a small goldfish bowl with a fish. The idea is to create energy that will cue you to move. These visual cues should be accompanied by hardware that enables you to move, such as a portable stepper beneath your desk and a cordless or long-cord phone.

NEAT BEAT: Pick a NEAT Project

Choose from one of these suggestions:

Draw a picture of your dream house.
Paint a picture of yourself and/or family.
Make a piece of clothing.
Make a piece of furniture (model or real).

In our culture of ready-made dinners and premoistened dusting cloths, few of us are forced to use our hands and our minds to make something anymore. Though it's nice to have the convenience, we lose our connection to the fundamental act of living when everything is handed to us in a disposable, ready-made package. We also lose a lot of NEAT. Today's NEAT Beat is a weeklong project that is designed to let you roll your sleeves up and tap into your tactile creativity. It may be tempting to just scribble a stick figure of yourself on a napkin and check the "done" box in your NEAT Planner. But please take your time and have fun with this. What you put in is what you get out. Your chosen project should make you think and dream. What would you put in your dream house? Walk around the neighborhood and notice the special features of houses you've always admired. Stop at a craft store and touch and feel all the amazing fabrics available to you. Even if you just make a scarf, you have created something out of your own imagination that is to your unique taste. Have fun with your self portrait. No one expects a Renoir. Use watercolors and create an impressionistic painting of yourself and your life. The spillover benefits aren't just greater NEAT, but also improved well-being. Research finds that expanding and building your creative sense helps you adapt to life with less stress by making you more flexible and open to new experience. And whatever you do, don't worry about how polished the end result looks. The benefits come from the process of setting your mind free to think and problem solve outside of its usual space, not from the actual product itself. Though I must say making your own shirt (which is what I did) does wonders for your confidence and self-esteem!

Though some of these activities, like knitting, may involve sitting, the act of gathering the materials definitely puts you on your feet. You also can increase the NEAT of each activity by standing to do it.

NEAT FUEL CELLS: Two-fuel-cell breakfast; two-fuel-cell lunch; two-fuel-cell dinner

This might be a good week to eat in more than you go out or take out. A study from Clemson University found that restaurant chefs typically serve up portions that are up to four times larger than those recommended by the USDA, even though more than three-quarters of them believe they're dishing out "regular" portions of food. Facing that much food can make following the fuel cell system nearly impossible, especially while you're still acclimating to eating appropriate amounts. If you must eat out, order appetizer portions or split the meal with a friend.

DAY 2 CHECKLIST: Today is a 6-point day

NEAT Feet: One twenty-minute walk; two thirty-minute walks. _____ / _____

NEAT Exercises: Ten Core Chargers and five Sunrise Stretches. _____
_____ points (3 points: 1 for *each* thirty-minute walk;
1 for the twenty-minute walk plus the NEAT exercises)

NEAT Beat: Pick a NEAT Project.
I choose to

_____.

Jot down a few notes about the NEAT Project you chose and
what you need to get it done.

_____

_____

_____

_____

_____

_____ points (2 points)

NEAT Fuel Cells: Two-fuel-cell breakfast; two-fuel-cell lunch; two-fuel-cell dinner. _____
_____ point (1 point for breakfast, lunch, and dinner)

Grand total: _____ (out of 6 points)

Day 3: Wednesday

NEAT FEET: One twenty-minute walk; two thirty-minute walks; ten Core Chargers and five Sunrise Stretches shortly after waking

If there's any activity more wonderful than walking, it would have to be dancing. It's virtually impossible to feel stressed or sad when you're moving to your favorite music. Shimmying and shaking to the beat is also remarkably good for you. In a study of eighty-eight men and women with heart disease, researchers found that those who danced for about twenty minutes three days a week for eight weeks improved their cardiovascular fitness by approximately 18 percent — just about the same as those who rode exercise bikes or walked on treadmills for the same amount of time. A similar study found that people who perform rhythmic exercise, like dancing, may significantly lower their levels of CRP (a protein in the blood that seems to raise the risk of heart disease), perhaps because people tend to dance for longer periods of time than they do formal exercise or because it lowers stress and makes them happy. One young female client listed "dancing to my iPod for 20 minutes a day" as one of her NEAT activity goals. It worked. She looked forward to taking a break in her day to tune out the world and groove. Even sashaying around the kitchen while you cook can do your body, and mind, a world of good.

NEAT BEAT: Assemble the supplies you need for your NEAT Project

As you start gathering the goods for your project, don't be surprised if you find yourself getting bitten by the creative hobby bug. Recent trends suggest that the NEAT play pendulum is starting to swing back into positive territory as people rediscover the joys of quilting, painting, knitting, pottery, model making, baking, and sewing. Even in San Francisco, the capital of high tech, the Stitch Lounge — an urban Starbucks-style sewing lounge where people can rent sewing machines by the hour — is bursting its seams with eager customers who, living in an electronics-saturated environment, are hungering for a NEAT outlet that is tactile and creative. After decades of free-falling, the number of sewing machines imported to the United States actually *doubled* from 1999 to 2005 as young people have taken a shine to sewing their own clothes for fun. It's living proof that NEAT can't be repressed for too long before people start pushing back, drawn by their biological yearnings to move and create. Even reality TV and YouTube give me hope. People are showing that they are no longer content to sit and watch and be passively entertained. They want to be part of the process.

NEAT FUEL CELLS: Two-fuel-cell breakfast; two-fuel-cell lunch; two-fuel-cell dinner; Slow-Food Wednesday

"But I really don't like vegetables!" I hear this lament with some frequency from clients who struggle to add plant foods to their plate. In reality, most people like *some* vegetables, even if it's just corn and occasionally carrots. If you turn green at the sight of spinach, do what millions of moms do for their finicky kids: Sneak them in. Shred carrots and zucchini and add them to pasta sauce; sauté sliced greens and blend them into burrito filling; mash steamed cauliflower and garlic along with potatoes. All those vegetables still count, even if you don't taste them!

DAY 3 CHECKLIST: Today is a 7-point day

NEAT Feet: One twenty-minute walk; two thirty-minute walks. ____/____

NEAT Exercises: Ten Core Chargers and five Sunrise Stretches. ____
____ points (3 points: 1 for *each* thirty-minute walk; 1 for the twenty-minute walk plus for the NEAT exercises)

NEAT Beat: Assemble the following supplies for my NEAT Project:

_____

_____

____ points (2 points)

NEAT Fuel Cells: Two-fuel-cell breakfast; two-fuel-cell lunch; two-fuel-cell dinner. ____
Slow-Food Wednesday. ____
____ points (2 points: 1 for breakfast, lunch, and dinner; 1 for no fast food)

Grand total: ____ (out of 7 points)

Day 4: Thursday

NEAT FEET: One twenty-minute walk; two thirty-minute walks; ten Core Chargers and five Sunrise Stretches shortly after waking

Do you own a treadmill yet? If not, it may be time to consider a purchase. It is a perfect way to get your daily NEAT while also enjoying your favorite shows. Because you're not running, you don't need to turn up the TV volume to unbearable levels. Since walking occupies you while you watch, you also don't have to worry about all that mindless snacking you might otherwise succumb to.

Concerned about the cost? It may also be time to investigate your priorities. Inevitably, when I have this discussion with clients, it goes something like this. Me: It would be great for you to have a treadmill. That way, you can get your NEAT no matter what the time, weather, or what favorite shows are on.

Client:	I can't afford one.
Me:	Do you have a high-definition TV?
Client:	Yes.
Me:	A treadmill costs considerably less.
Client:	Well, we don't have room.
Me:	What do you watch TV on?

Client: A La-Z-Boy.

You get the picture. I'm not suggesting you take out a second mortgage and replace your furniture with exercise equipment. But you can get a quality treadmill for less than $1,000. You can save that much by eating out less and socking away $100 a month. You can also find many perfectly functional secondhand models on eBay or at www.freecycle.org. I bought mine for $350, and it's still going strong three years later. I "trash picked" my stationary bike, and it's still in perfect working condition. As to the treadmill placement, you won't use it if you stick it in a dark corner of the basement. Rearrange the furniture a bit and make it part of the entertainment room, so everyone will be inspired to hop on and increase their NEAT. It's an investment in your family's health and well-being.

When shopping for a treadmill, there are a few essentials: Measure the space where you plan to put it before you go to the store. Showrooms are big, which always make the machines look smaller than they really are. Test-drive each machine for at least ten to fifteen minutes before you buy. It should feel smooth and stable and be relatively quiet, so you can watch TV without turning the volume to unreasonable decibel levels. The treadmill should come with at least a one-year, on-site warranty, and there should be a local service network available to come fix the machine should it need repair. Don't be sold on any fancy features like heart-rate monitoring and programming that you likely won't use. Stick to the basics — time, speed, and distance — and you can save money and still go home with a solid machine.

If your living space is small and you don't have room for a treadmill, do consider one of the portable steppers mentioned earlier. As a bonus, you can even carry it from room to room to use it wherever you are! Or, if cost is the issue, consider putting an exercise bike in front of the TV. You can find secondhand bikes for next to nothing at yard sales, secondhand stores, and eBay.

NEAT BEAT: Work on your NEAT Project

If you haven't already, dig in today. Unless you're making something intricate like a dress or a dresser (in which case, I give you a hearty round of applause!), you should be able to finish your project by Sunday. Make that your goal.

Also, plan a Sunday NEAT activity. As you do, make a concerted effort to be decisive. When Joe, a thirty-five-year-old copy editor with about 10 pounds to lose, first read all my recommendations, he bristled. "This all takes a lot of planning. I don't want to think about what I'm doing Sunday when it's only Thursday. I can figure out Sunday on Sunday." And therein lied the problem. Sunday would come, and because he had failed to plan, the day would slip away, and before he knew it, he'd done nothing. That would be okay if Joe were happy about doing nothing; in reality, however, he wanted to do *something,* but he just didn't figure it out until it was too late. Sound familiar? How often do you find yourself in a similar situation? You figure you'll do something big and fun or productive on the weekend, but you don't plan for it. So you sleep in, read the paper, putter around, and then feel sad and dissatisfied that it's three in the afternoon and nothing's been done. By planning just one thing, you actually get more done, because it puts you in motion and gives you a focal point around which to plan other activities.

For instance, let's say you plan to go to the zoo with your family. You can plan on being there when the doors open and spending the two or so hours it takes to walk around the grounds. Then, maybe an IKEA store is on the way home. So you plan to stop there and pick up some supplies for one of your long-standing home improvement projects. Then you come home and, excited by your new purchases, begin organizing that home improvement project. Joe, who incidentally did start planning (and lost those 10 pounds), found this out firsthand. "The best part is that once I planned my active time, I found I could also plan my downtime," he said. "I would plan a project in the morning that I planned to wrap up by early afternoon, so I could watch a football game — guilt-free!"

Start by checking your local paper for weekend activities in your area (most papers post these by Thursday). Then plan away. Try something completely different.

- Find a local orchard and go berry, apple, or pumpkin picking.
- Check out the new galleries at a local museum.
- Organize a touch football game with your friends and their families.
- Go to a lake or river nearby and rent a kayak or canoe for the morning.
- Ride along a trail or bike path.
- Go bird watching.
- Visit your local historical center and learn something new about your town.
- Attend a craft show, flea market, or farmers' market.

NEAT FUEL CELLS: Two-fuel-cell breakfast; two-fuel-cell lunch; two-fuel-cell dinner; no second helpings today

When it comes to food, there is definitely a law of diminishing returns. The first few bites of any good meal are always the most delectable. Then, though the food may still be as good, the subsequent bites are less scrumptious. Without fail, the second helping of a dish is never, ever as satisfying as the first. That's why I added the no-second-helping rule to today's NEAT Eat. I want you to slow down and enjoy your food. There's a saying in restaurant circles: You take the first bite with your eyes. Take care to present your food in an attractive fashion. Put it on a plate. Garnish it with some sliced tomatoes. Sprinkle it with a colorful vinegar. Then slow down and savor every bite. When you're done, get up from the table and put your dishes in the sink. Go do something else for ten to fifteen minutes to see if you truly are still hungry. If you are, don't go back and get more of the same food. Find something sweet, such as mandarin orange slices or berries with a little cream, to finish the meal on a satisfying note. Make this a daily habit.

DAY 4 CHECKLIST: Today is a 6-point day

NEAT Feet: One twenty-minute walk; two thirty-minute walks. _____/_____

NEAT Exercises: Ten Core Chargers and five Sunrise Stretches. _____
_____ points (3 points: 1 for *each* thirty-minute walk;
1 for the twenty-minute walk plus for the NEAT exercises)

NEAT Beat: Report progress on my NEAT Project.

_____

_____

_____

On Sunday, I am going to
_____.
I selected this because:

_____

_____

_____ point (1 point)

_____

NEAT Fuel Cells: Two-fuel-cell breakfast; two-fuel-cell lunch; two-fuel-cell dinner. ____
No second helpings. ____
____ points (2 points: 1 for breakfast, lunch, and dinner; 1 for no second helpings)

Grand total: ____ (out of 6 points)

Day 5: Friday

NEAT FEET: One twenty-minute walk; two thirty-minute walks; ten Core Chargers and five Sunrise Stretches shortly after waking

Are you enjoying yourself? Though this will sometimes feel like work as you become accustomed to living in a whole new way, it is supposed to be fun. If it's not, you will never stick to it. That's why I want to make sure you are getting maximum pleasure from every step you take. Today, write down five things that would make your walking more fun. Stumped? Here are some suggestions.

- **Listen to a story.** Reading is a tremendously pleasurable and important activity, and I would never suggest swapping your books for earbuds. But you can enjoy even more literature by listening to some of it via books on tape. Most libraries (remember the library?) have a wide selection you can borrow, and they'll make your walking time fly by. (As with any handheld technology, you should only listen to books while you walk when you're in a completely safe environment.)

- **Go somewhere.** It's hard to overemphasize this one. You will love your walks so much more when they take you somewhere, whether it's a friend's house, a store, or your favorite espresso shop.
- **Get a dog.** A recent survey of households in British Columbia found that dog owners spent an average of 300 minutes a week — that's about 43 minutes a day — in mild to moderate activity (including walking the dog, playing with the dog, and grooming the dog). Those without canine companions averaged only 168 minutes. Plus, pets lower blood pressure and enhance your enjoyment of life.
- **Pick some podcasts.** You can download most of your favorite radio shows for free. Or go to a site like iTunes and check out the wide array of podcasts that will enrich your NEAT walking. You'll find news, sports, entertainment, and in-

terviews — even podcasts for learning a new language.

- **Return with a story.** A friend of mine makes it a point to tell her six-year-old boy all the new things she saw on her daily walk. Sometimes they're exciting, like the time she saw a small herd of deer eating apples from a neighbor's tree. Other times, they're small or amusing, like seeing squirrels chasing each other up a tree or noting a house on the corner that is still all decked out for Christmas though it's long past Easter. This simple ritual forces her to be in the moment, taking in her surroundings, deepening her connection with her son, and teaching him the wonders of walking.

NEAT BEAT: Work on your NEAT Project

Confirm the details of your Sunday plan. Tie up loose ends today. Check that your NEAT Project will be done by Sunday and that Sunday's plans are gelled, so all you need to do is get up and go. Remember, NEAT planning is central to NEAT living. It only takes a few seconds, so do it!

NEAT FUEL CELLS: Two-fuel-cell breakfast; two-fuel-cell lunch; two-fuel-cell dinner; Fat-free Friday

We haven't looked too closely at the liquid part of your diet yet, but we will in the upcoming weeks. One of the beverages that always comes up is coffee. My patients frequently ask (with fingers firmly crossed, I'm sure) if coffee is "bad" for them, or if they can continue to enjoy their daily java fix(es) while following the NEAT Plan. A major scientific analysis published in the *New England Journal of Medicine* concluded that coffee appears to be quite safe. A growing body of evidence shows that your favorite morning pick-me-up is actually good for you. Researchers from the University of Scranton found that coffee is the number one source of antioxidants in the American diet. Also, aside from keeping you alert and awake, coffee appears to provide protection against type 2 diabetes, liver cancer, colon cancer, and Parkinson's disease. Of course, going overboard (especially if you're not a coffee drinker) can leave you jittery and cause stomach upset, so be sensible about your Starbucks visits (remember the chart on page 189). Speaking of coffee, we're talking plain coffee with maybe a bit of milk and sugar here, not a whipped cream, sugar-syrup-laden concoction. (Remember, a Frappuccino can have more calories than a two-fuel-cell meal!) Keep it simple and enjoy it to your heart's content.

DAY 5 CHECKLIST: Today is a 7-point day

NEAT Feet: One twenty-minute walk; two thirty-minute walks. _____/_____

NEAT Exercises: Ten Core Chargers and five Sunrise Stretches. _____ _____ points (3 points: 1 for *each* thirty-minute walk; 1 for the twenty-minute walk plus for the NEAT exercises)

NEAT Beat: Report progress on my NEAT Project.

_____

_____

_____

_____

On Sunday, I am going to _____.
Hours of operation:
_____.
Location:
_____.
Plan for the day (when you'll leave, what you'll do):
_____

_____ points (2 points)

NEAT Fuel Cells: Two-fuel-cell breakfast; two-fuel-cell lunch; two-fuel-cell dinner.

_____
Fat-free Friday. _____
_____ points (2 points: 1 for breakfast, lunch, and dinner; 1 for going fat-free)

Grand total: _____ (out of 7 points)

Day 6: Saturday

NEAT FEET: One twenty-minute walk; two thirty-minute walks; ten Core Chargers and five Sunrise Stretches shortly after waking

There's a woman in my neighborhood for whom I have the utmost admiration. Every morning, without fail, regardless of the weather, she is out there walking (and often talking on her cell phone). I once asked her how she did it. Wasn't she ever deterred by the rain or snow? "Oh, I have walking outfits for every condition. So I just check the weather the night before and lay out what I'm going to wear. That way, I'm prepared and not surprised or put off by the weather. I just suit up and go." This is clearly why she is so slim, strong, and vibrant, well into her mid-sixties.

It may take some trial and error at first, but with just a few key pieces of clothing, you can be prepared for whatever Mother Nature brings your way. The most important tenet of dressing for the weather is layering. To stay warm during chilly weather walks, you're better off wearing multiple layers rather than trying to wear a single thick one. Layers trap your body heat between them, so you stay warmer. You can also remove a layer should the temperatures rise unexpectedly. A light, easy-to-open jacket that provides wind and rain protection should always be your top layer. And don't forget a hat and gloves. When your head and hands are warm, so is the rest of you.

NEAT BEAT: Plan to showcase your NEAT Project

Be proud of your project! It's something you've crafted with your own two hands out of your own imagination. Today, as you finish it up, plan how you're going to show it off. If it's an article of clothing, wear it to work on Monday (or at least out on Sunday afternoon). If it's a picture, frame it. Pick a spot to display your model, if that's what you made. It should be a reminder of what is possible when you put your mind — and NEAT energy — to work. Also as part of today's NEAT Beat, see today's NEAT Fuel Cell guide and examine the reasons you eat.

NEAT FUEL CELLS: Two-fuel-cell breakfast; two-fuel-cell lunch; two-fuel-cell dinner

Take an emotional inventory today. My clients who struggle while following the eating plan are those who are emotional eaters. They're accustomed to eating when they're happy, sad, stressed, or angry. Not being able to use food for comfort or reward leads to more emotions, which in turn sharpens the urge to eat. Hopefully, your NEAT Feet and NEAT Beats are keeping you sufficiently occupied, so the emotional food cravings are not too overwhelming. If they are, you may need to work on some calming strategies to cool these cravings. One that my clients find works best is remarkably simple. Acknowledge your urges to eat for what they are. Tell yourself, "I'm not really hungry. I want to eat because my boss overloaded me with work today and I didn't meet my NEAT Feet quota." Then turn to another activity for stress relief. Now tell yourself, "Okay, I'm not going to eat for emotional reasons, because that always just makes me feel worse in the end. Instead, I will take a long walk." Or you can tackle a home improvement project or play with your kids. Whatever you choose, *say it out loud to yourself.* Then do it. The best part is that you'll be rewarded twice: once with the instant gratification of checking off a NEAT activity and racking up points, and again with your eventual weight loss.

DAY 6 CHECKLIST: Today is a 6-point day

NEAT Feet: One twenty-minute walk; two thirty-minute walks. ____ / ____

NEAT Exercises: Ten Core Chargers and five Sunrise Stretches. ____
____ points (3 points: 1 for *each* thirty-minute walk;
1 for the twenty-minute walk plus for the NEAT exercises)

NEAT Beat: Made plans to showcase my NEAT Project. ____
The top three emotional reasons I eat:

_____

_____

_____ points (2 points)

NEAT Fuel Cells: Two-fuel-cell breakfast; two-fuel-cell lunch; two-fuel-cell dinner.

_____ point (1 point for breakfast, lunch, and dinner)

Grand total: _____ (out of 6 points)

Saturday is weigh-in day: Weigh yourself in the morning and jot the number here. _____

Day 7: Sunday

NEAT FEET: One twenty-minute walk; two 30-minute walks; ten Core Chargers and five Sunrise Stretches shortly after waking

Sock it to your feet! Nearly as important as comfortable walking shoes are supportive, well-fitting socks. Your socks are the first line of defense against the pressure, rubbing, and sweat that can lead to discomfort, hot spots, or blisters. Believe it or not, there are socks specifically designed for walking, and I highly recommend picking up a few pairs. What makes a quality walking sock? For one, the material. You want wicking fabrics such as COOLMAX, merino wool, Dri-FIT, bamboo, or Sorbtek. Cotton tends to hold moisture, so steer clear of all-cotton socks. Walking socks should hug your feet comfortably, so they don't bunch up or slip down. If you tend to get sore feet, also look for socks with padding in the ball and heel of the foot. They will cushion those strike points so you can walk in comfort.

NEAT BEAT: Execute your planned NEAT activity

Have a brilliant day today! It is crucial to appreciate that if your NEAT activity involves you being on your legs, it counts toward your NEAT Feet. So if your NEAT activity today is going to the art gallery and you did it for two hours, you get 2 points for completing the NEAT Beat *plus* 2 points for completing your NEAT Feet. That's 4 points at one shot. Way to go!

NEAT FUEL CELLS: Two-fuel-cell breakfast; two-fuel-cell lunch; two-fuel-cell dinner; Cook-Something Sunday

Remember, Sunday is cooking day on the NEAT Plan. If you haven't already started making a habit out of cooking something every Sunday, now is the time. This is a tremendous opportunity to set the stage for healthy eating all week long. Roast a chicken to eat in sandwiches at lunch. Make a big pot of soup. Keep it simple with basic fresh ingredients.

DAY 7 CHECKLIST: Today is a 7-point day

NEAT Feet: One twenty-minute walk; two thirty-minute walks. _____/_____

NEAT Exercises: Ten Core Chargers and five Sunrise Stretches. _____

You've just logged twenty-one days in a row of walking. Congratulations on your new healthy habit!

_____ points (3 points: 1 for *each* thirty-minute walk;
1 for the twenty-minute walk plus for the NEAT exercises)

NEAT Beat: How did your planned NEAT activity go? What would you do the same? Differently?

_____

_____

_____

_____ points (2 points)

_____

_____

NEAT Fuel Cells: Two-fuel-cell breakfast; two-fuel-cell lunch; two-fuel-cell dinner. _____

Cook-Something Sunday. _____ _____ points (2 points: 1 for breakfast, lunch, and dinner; 1 for cooking something)

_____

_____

Grand total: _____ (out of 7 points)

_____

END-OF-WEEK ADD-UP

Maximum points: 46
My points: _____

10
WEEK 4: MIND YOUR BODY

Contrary to how you may view yourself, your body is more than a life support system for your mind, and your mind affects much more than your thoughts. They are inextricably connected. What one does profoundly affects the other. It's common knowledge that doctors sometimes prescribe placebos (sugar pills) — not because they think patients are dumb, but because they know that your mind can make you healthy as well as it can make you ill. Likewise, when your body gets injured, the mind often suffers in the form of depression and anxiety. Your movement affects your brain chemicals, and your brain chemicals affect your movement. Mental health, I believe, is the most profound argument for NEAT. Sedentary living leads to physical immobility through overweight and poor fitness, which leads to mental lethargy and depression.

This week's NEAT Beats are devoted to

helping you rediscover (or perhaps discover for the first time) your body-mind relationship. We'll extend and expand your NEAT Feet, so they branch into even more aspects of your life. And we'll look at alcohol (a mind-body drug if there ever was one) intake, as well as snacking, as part of this week's NEAT fueling. As you forge a deeper connection between mind and body, you'll quickly find that living an active life carries benefits that far exceed weight loss or improved physical health.

Day 1: Monday

NEAT FEET: Three thirty-minute walks; twenty Core Chargers and eight Sunrise Stretches shortly after waking

Note the bump in all three elements of your NEAT Feet today. You're walking a little longer, allowing your feet to take you even farther. You're also doing twice as many Core Chargers and a few more Sunrise Stretches. The fitter and stronger you are, the easier it will be to be of sound body *and* mind on your NEAT journey. These additions will take no more than another few minutes in your day, but they will reward you with quality years in your life.

NEAT BEAT: Name a person whose work you

admire (can be anyone in any field: musician, politician, scientist, activist, artist, writer, actor, sports star)

We have a tendency to view the successful people we admire as somehow luckier than we are. We think they must be smarter or have had more opportunities or just found the road to success easier than us. That is very rarely the case. In most cases, they tried and often failed many times to reach their high tier of achievement. They just kept moving forward. It's all part of the NEAT journey. Today, take a few minutes to research the person you've chosen. Then fill out the following questionnaire.

Person's name: _____

What was his/her maximum education level? _____

Who were his/her principal influences/mentors en route to success?

_____

What barriers did he/she overcome to become successful (e.g., his/her first record sold seven copies; tried to become a senator four times before being elected)

What would you have done if faced with those barriers? _____

_____

_____

How can you apply his/her lessons to your own life? _____

_____

_____

_____

NEAT FUEL CELLS: Two-fuel-cell breakfast; two-fuel-cell lunch; two-fuel-cell dinner; NEAT-Fuel Snack Challenge

Time to tackle the final piece of NEAT fueling — snacking. It is common to snack for many reasons that have absolutely nothing to do with hunger. Boredom, stress, procrastination, even happiness can send us sailing to the refrigerator or vending machine for some therapy, comfort, or reward. Take a few minutes to evaluate your own snack attacks. What usually drives them? (*Note:* If it is truly hunger, that's legitimate; write it down.)

_____

_____

_____

What is your very favorite snack? (Pick the one that you eat most often. Cheesecake doesn't count if you only have it once a year. M&M's do if you have them nearly every day.)

_____

This week's NEAT-Fuel Snack Challenge is to go a full week without that snack. This is not meant to be punishing or cruel. It is intended to make you think about what you're snacking on and why. If you can't automatically reach for the bag of chips, you'll have to think about what else you want, which will lead you to examine more closely what void the snack is filling, whether it be real hunger or emotional hunger.

DAY 1 CHECKLIST: Today is a 7-point day

NEAT Feet: Three thirty-minute walks.
_____/_____/_____

NEAT Exercises: Twenty Core Chargers and eight Sunrise Stretches. _____ _____ points (3 points: 2 for the three walks; 1 for the NEAT exercises)

NEAT Beat: Identified a person I admire and filled out questionnaire. _____ Jot a few notes about what you learned that surprised you (about your person or yourself).

_____

_____

_____ points (2 points)

NEAT Fuel Cells: Two-fuel-cell breakfast; two-fuel-cell lunch; two-fuel-cell dinner.

_____

Agreed to NEAT-Fuel Snack Challenge.

_____

_____ points (2 points: 1 for breakfast, lunch, and
dinner; 1 for the NEAT-Fuel Snack
Challenge)

Grand total: _____ (out of 7 points)

Day 2: Tuesday

**NEAT FEET: Three thirty-minute walks; twenty
Core Chargers and eight Sunrise Stretches
shortly after waking**

My clients often ask if they should buy a
pedometer. Although I generally encourage anything used to promote NEAT, I
usually caution my patients against relying
too heavily on these step counters. When
you look at how normal people spend their
days, the average speed of walking is about
1 mile per hour. This includes flicking

through clothes on the clothes rack, strolling down to lunch, walking to the bathroom, and sometimes running for a bus. The true average of all of those walks is 1 mile per hour. When you look at the accuracy of over-the-counter pedometers at this speed, they are abysmal. Their accuracy is about 30 percent, and what they report is inconsistent. That means if you set your "step goal" at 10,000 steps, as is often recommended, the pedometer may say you've reached this goal when you've actually fallen far short. Likewise (and often more disheartening), the pedometer may read 7,000 steps, but you have actually walked 11,000. The larger trouble is that step counting does not focus on living an active, engaged life in which you stand instead of sit, hang shelving instead of watch TV, and call a loved one rather than sit and surf the Internet, but rather focuses you on looking at numbers. This can be a distraction, since the essence of NEAT living is in the fun of doing it. If you love gadgets and find them motivating, I would encourage you to investigate the Gruve NEAT-monitoring device described on page 164. It was specifically designed to monitor NEAT activity, so it will be more accurate and ultimately motivating.

NEAT BEAT: What has helped you? What has hurt you?

We all have turning points in life, experiences that propel us toward our goals or that knock us off track . . . or worse, backward. Many people don't give them much thought after they happen; but they're important to acknowledge, especially the bad episodes, because they can linger and continue blocking your progress for many years after the fact. Likewise, the good experiences can help you overcome these obstacles if you draw strength from them, which is today's mission.

Write down three positive experiences that made you stronger or helped you be more successful.

_____

_____

_____

Write down three negative experiences that set you back or prevented you from reaching your goals and dreams.

_____

_____

_____

Note: This exercise may stir up buried, negative feelings. That is okay. To make real progress, you need to acknowledge the impact those experiences had on you. As we move forward, the goal is to minimize these experiences and push past them. If getting past these negative experiences is impossible for you, please put the plan on hold and talk to a professional (many churches offer free counseling programs). Your local library will have resources as well. This is where your feet need to take you today. Confronting this pain and the impact it has had on your life is the only way to move forward.

NEAT FUEL CELLS: Two-fuel-cell breakfast; two-fuel-cell lunch; two-fuel-cell dinner; continue the NEAT-Fuel Snack Challenge

Like all of NEAT fueling, successful NEAT snacking takes planning. If you wait until you are famished or completely stressed to figure out your afternoon snack, you're doomed to grab the most gooey, fat-laden sugar bomb within arm's reach. Don't let that happen. Create three one-fuel-cell (200-calorie) snacks that will satisfy your hunger and urge to eat without weighing you down (mentally and physically). Here are some easy options my clients enjoy.

1 packet of instant oatmeal (low sugar) topped with berries

- Apple slices with a tablespoon of peanut butter
- 6 ounces of yogurt (plain) drizzled with honey or maple syrup and sprinkled with cinnamon
- 3 slices mini pumpernickel or Wasa bread, with one slice cheese
- 4 whole grain crackers smeared with nut butter
- 1 crunchy granola bar
- 2 fig bars, for when you crave something sweet
- 20 baked tortilla chips with salsa

Plan what you'll eat and when. "I used to just let my snacking happen," said Mary, who has lost a pound per week on the NEAT Plan. "But then it would just happen and happen and happen without me even thinking about it. Now I plan to have a specific snack at 3 p.m. It's great! I'm not distracted thinking about food. I know I'll eat at 3. And I'm satisfied because I ate a planned snack instead of just nibbling here and there."

DAY 2 CHECKLIST: Today is a 7-point day

NEAT Feet: Three thirty-minute walks.

_____/_____/_____

NEAT Exercises: Twenty Core Chargers
and eight
Sunrise Stretches. _____
_____ points (3 points: 2 for the three
walks;
1 for the NEAT exercises)

NEAT Beat: Listed my positive and
negative experiences.
_____

If needed, I will talk to someone to
overcome barriers from any overwhelming
negative experiences.
Please note below who you talk to and
when. Don't hesitate.
Call today, if you need some extra help.

_____

_____

_____ points (2 points)

NEAT Fuel Cells: Two-fuel-cell breakfast;
two-fuel-cell lunch; two-fuel-cell dinner.
_____

Bought/made one-fuel-cell snack. _____
How did you feel about forgoing your
favorite snack today?

What snacks did you have instead?

_____

_____

_____ points (2 points: 1 for breakfast, lunch, and dinner; 1 for NEAT-Fuel Snack Challenge)

Grand total: _____ (out of 7 points)

Day 3: Wednesday

NEAT FEET: Three thirty-minute walks; twenty Core Chargers and eight Sunrise Stretches shortly after waking

Listening to music when you walk may help you walk farther and lose more weight. In a study of forty-one overweight women, researchers at Fairleigh Dickinson University found that those who listened to music while they walked lost twice as much weight (16 pounds) and body fat (4 percent) over the twenty-four-week study than those who took their steps in silence. If music motivates you and you take your treks in safe, well-populated areas, by all means, plug in your iPod and boogie down the street.

NEAT BEAT: Stop by the supermarket and buy

315

some Play-Doh or clay (you'll see why tomor-row)

Today, plan a NEAT activity for Saturday. If possible, connect this activity to the person you admire. If Leonardo da Vinci tops your list, take the family to a science museum or even go out for a family bike ride (some say da Vinci was the first to sketch a modern bike). If it was a musician, check out some live music or, even better, schedule time to play some of your own. Maybe you won't ever be an accomplished pianist or a renowned physicist, but you can always expand your knowledge and broaden your expertise. By exploring and enjoying the realm of your role models, you can reignite your own creative spark, which will bring you that much closer to realizing your own goals and potential.

On Saturday, I am going to _____.

I selected this because:

_____

_____

_____

NEAT FUEL CELLS: Two-fuel-cell breakfast; two-fuel-cell lunch; two-fuel-cell dinner; one-fuel-cell snack; Slow-Food Wednesday

If you haven't already done so, today is the

day to start applying the fuel cell rules to your snacks. Each snack is one fuel cell. You can spread your snacks out during the day, enjoying one midmorning and one midafternoon or one midafternoon and one in the evening. Or you can add one fuel cell to a meal, like lunch, so lunch now becomes a three-cell meal. Experiment a little to find the configuration that fuels you best. Some of my patients find smaller bits of food throughout the day sustain them better than "three squares" (or fuel cells, as the case may be). Others like to sit down to a larger plate of food less frequently. And always remember that carrots, apples, and other fruits and veggies are yours to enjoy without keeping track of them. Enjoy your seven fuel cells your way.

DAY 3 CHECKLIST: Today is a 6-point day

NEAT Feet: Three thirty-minute walks. ____/____/____

NEAT Exercises: Twenty Core Chargers and eight Sunrise Stretches. ____
____ points (3 points: 2 for the three walks; 1

for the NEAT exercises)

NEAT Beat: On Saturday, I am going
to _____.
Hours of operation:
_____.
Location:
_____.
Plan for the day (i.e., when you'll leave,
what you'll do):

_____

_____

_____

_____ point (1 point)

NEAT Fuel Cells: Two-fuel-cell breakfast;
two-fuel-cell lunch;
two-fuel-cell dinner; one-fuel-cell snack.

_____
Slow-Food Wednesday. _____
_____ points (2 points: 1 for breakfast,
lunch, dinner, and
snack; 1 for no fast food)

Grand total: _____ (out of 6 points)

Day 4: Thursday

NEAT FEET: Three thirty-minute walks; twenty Core Chargers and eight Sunrise Stretches shortly after waking

At this point, you should be working your NEAT Feet seamlessly into your day, using the time to actually go somewhere and accomplish daily tasks. Keep your walks fresh through constant exploration. Albert Einstein argued that we become defined by the spaces we inhabit. When you're confined to a chair, you become sedentary in your mind. You've liberated yourself from that fate. But avoid falling into the rut of always going to the same places down the same paths. Walk down new streets. Explore new avenues. Check out new stores, galleries, parks, and shopping centers. The more you open yourself to environmental stimuli, the more creative and regenerated you'll feel. Your destination is limited only by the direction you choose to go.

"We've discovered there's more within walking distance from us than we realized," said Lisa, a mother of three, who now weighs what she did in college. "There's a restaurant we like that's a mile away. When my husband and I have a date night, we now walk there and back."

NEAT BEAT: Mold your experience

Go back to your list of bad experiences you wrote down on Tuesday. Now take your clay or Play-Doh and mold an object that represents any aspect of that experience. Maybe it's a wall that represents the time you got passed over for a promotion. Or a target that represents how you felt when you got fired. Or a broken heart for how it felt when your partner left you. Whatever it is, mold it to the best of your ability and place it on a shelf until tomorrow.

Remember your NEAT Goals and dreams? Confronting our obstacles is a huge step in reaching them. Don't be surprised if you find yourself uncomfortable with this process. For many of us, our obstacles are actually our safety nets, convenient excuses for not trying to reach our dreams and something to fall back on if we miss. Carl Jung said our dreams are actually the things we fear most! I have found that to be quite true. We are afraid to confront what we really want because it takes hard work and movement out of our familiar comfort zone to get it. By embarking on the NEAT journey, you're already moving out of your comfort zone. Now, bit by little bit, we'll do the hard work to remove obstacles, confront fears, and take you another step closer to your dream life.

Today, also plan a NEAT activity for Saturday. (It's important to keep planning; we don't do what we don't plan.)

NEAT FUEL CELLS: Two-fuel-cell breakfast; two-fuel-cell lunch; two-fuel-cell dinner; one-fuel-cell snack

When archaeologists discovered beer jugs dating back to the Stone Age, they established the fact that humankind has always enjoyed a good drink. Intentionally fermented beverages have existed at least as early as the Neolithic period (ca. 10,000 BC), and some scientists believe that beer may have preceded bread as a staple in the caveman kitchen. Alcohol is a part of modern living. A little bit of alcohol — say, a drink per day a few days per week — is perfectly healthy. More is not. Too much can have serious short- and long-term consequences. How much alcohol do you drink? If you don't keep track, it's time to start. Though it makes you feel giddy at first, alcohol is a depressant, which means it slows your central nervous system function. You're more likely to eat too much and less likely to be productive when you're drinking, which makes too much alcohol incompatible with active, fully engaged NEAT living.

Starting today, write down the number of

alcoholic drinks you consume. Remember, one drink is considerably less than most people think. One standard drink is technically any drink that contains 14 grams of alcohol. That equals:

12 ounces of beer
5 ounces of wine
1.5 ounces of liquor

If you drink mixed drinks, drink draft beer, or use goblet style wineglasses, there's a really good chance you're getting more than one standard drink per beverage. Measure out the proper amount of alcohol at home to get a sense for what one drink looks and feels like. Alcohol has calories and those calories count. For the NEAT Plan, each drink is one-half of a fuel cell from here on out.

Also, ask yourself the hard question: Am I drinking too much?

The answer is yes, if you are:

A woman who has more than seven drinks per week or more than three drinks per occasion.

A man who has more than fourteen drinks per week or more than four drinks per occasion.

If that describes you, scale back on your weekly alcohol intake or seek help from your health-care provider.

DAY 4 CHECKLIST: Today is a 7-point day

NEAT Feet: Three thirty-minute walks.
_____/_____/_____

NEAT Exercises: Twenty Core Chargers and eight Sunrise Stretches.

_____

_____ points (3 points: 2 for the three walks; 1 for the NEAT exercises)

NEAT Beat: Made a mold of my bad experience. _____
Jot down a few notes on what you created and what it symbolizes.

_____

_____

_____

_____

_____

My NEAT activity for Saturday will be:

_____

_____

_____

_____

_____

_____ points (2 points)

_____

NEAT Fuel Cells: Two-fuel-cell breakfast; two-fuel-cell lunch; two-fuel-cell dinner; one-fuel-cell snack. _____
Number of alcoholic drinks I had today.

_____

_____ points (2 points: 1 for breakfast, lunch, dinner, and snack; 1 for tallying up alcoholic drinks)

_____

Grand total: _____ (out of 7 points)

Day 5: Friday

NEAT FEET: Three thirty-minute walks; twenty Core Chargers and eight Sunrise Stretches shortly after waking

Whenever I ask modern office workers to identify the biggest stresses in their jobs, e-mail inevitably ranks high on the list. How can a technological miracle that so simplifies communication be such a large source of stress? Because it exceeds the natural pace of human interaction. There is no silence or space for thought. I was speaking at an average-sized company in Missouri about the role of sedentary living and work on our health. At one point, I flippantly said, "I bet you couldn't live a day without e-mail." The vice president shot up from his chair as if electrified by 20,000 volts. "That's brilliant!" he said. I initially assumed he was being sarcastic — but he meant it. The company survived on product innovation, and he had long believed that creativity was being stifled by what he called "tic-tac" interactions. "You know," he said to me, "no one thinks anymore — we just respond." He instituted e-mail-free Fridays effective immediately. People loved it. "We actually talk," raved one worker. "I walk when I used to just e-mail her," noted another. "I'm so much more productive, I leave an hour earlier on Friday," said one man. The notion of e-mail-free Friday was not to divest people of an incredibly powerful technology, but rather to educate people how to apply it in the most effective way. Try it yourself and see what happens. If it's impossible to go e-mail free for a day, then check e-mail just twice a day: once before lunch, once late in the afternoon. Get up and respond to those messages you can. Reply to the rest the usual way. You'll still move more and be more productive.

NEAT BEAT: Shape your future

Take your molding from yesterday and re-shape it into something positive and new. Like your negative sculpture, the new one should be symbolic of the life you want to fashion for yourself. It might be a ladder that symbolizes upward mobility on your job. Or a palm tree that represents where you'd like to live. Again, mold it to the best of your ability. Then place it somewhere you'll see it every day.

As you're reshaping your negative model into a positive sculpture, make a promise to yourself that you will put that bad experience behind you. (It might be cathartic to take your fist and pound the negative sculpture completely flat before giving it its new and improved shape.) Whatever happened, whoever was to blame, whatever you or anyone else did, it's done. Over. In the past. You must forgive it and move forward. Many people struggle with forgiveness, especially when they feel they've been wronged, but as one of my colleagues in the mental-health division at Mayo Clinic explains, forgiveness is merely the act of untying yourself from the thoughts and feelings that bind you to the offense committed against you or that you committed. This doesn't mean you're forgetting or condoning it. You're simply reducing the power these feelings have over you, so you can live a freer, happier, more NEAT life. In 1600, Descartes described how your present divides your past from your future. Your future is yours to mold, starting today.

NEAT FUEL CELLS: Two-fuel-cell breakfast; two-fuel-cell lunch; two-fuel-cell dinner; one-fuel-cell snack; Fat-free Friday

While you're watching your alcoholic drinks this week, keep an eye on your other fluid intake as well. Researchers from the University of North Carolina at Chapel Hill have strong evidence that how much we drink has a strong relationship to how much we weigh. In a study of the drinking patterns of more than 46,500 adults between 1965 and 2002, the researchers found that during these thirty-seven years, though the amount of water drank stayed roughly the same, the number of calories Americans consumed from other beverages nearly doubled. Drinks such as juice, tea, soda, beer, and specialty coffee beverages now account for 21 percent of our daily calorie intake, up from just 12 percent in 1977. The problem is that beverages don't fill you up. They're just added energy, often in the form of empty calories. Diet sodas don't seem to be the answer, either. According to a study published in *Physiology & Behavior,* dieters who drink them regularly have higher body mass indexes than those who don't. If you've gotten in the habit of drinking all day, pick up a reusable stainless steel bottle, fill it with water and a dash of lemon juice for flavor, and take it with you wherever you go.

DAY 5 CHECKLIST: Today is a 7-point day

NEAT Feet: Three thirty-minute walks.
_____/_____/_____

NEAT Exercises: Twenty Core Chargers and eight Sunrise Stretches. _____

_____ points (3 points: 2 for the three walks;
1 for the NEAT exercises)

NEAT Beat: Created a positive future sculpture. _____

Jot down a few notes on what you
created and what it symbolizes.

_____

_____

_____

_____

_____ points (2 points)

_____

_____

NEAT Fuel Cells: Two-fuel-cell breakfast;
two-fuel-cell lunch;
two-fuel-cell dinner; one-fuel-cell snack.

_____

Fat-free Friday. _____
Number of alcoholic drinks I had today.

_____

_____ points (2 points: 1 for breakfast,
lunch, dinner,
and snack; 1 for Fat-free Friday)

_____

_____

Grand total: _____ (out of 7 points)

_____

Day 6: Saturday
NEAT FEET: Three thirty-minute walks; one
fifteen-minute walk; twenty Core Chargers and
eight Sunrise Stretches shortly after waking
Yes, we've added a fourth NEAT Feet

today. But remember, this is supposed to fit into your life, not take time away from it. It is crucial to remember that any activity that involves you being on your legs for any amount of time counts as a NEAT Feet. So if you decide to go shopping at the Mall of America (or whatever mall is closest to you) and you are out there on your feet for two hours, you're done!

NEAT BEAT: Perform your NEAT activity

"It's so fun to be an active person!" said my client Nancy one day. She had lost 10 pounds, but to her that was just the icing on the cake. What she really loved was how NEAT living made her feel so *alive*. "Over the years, with getting married and having kids and working hard on my job, I had gradually become really sedentary without even noticing it," she recalled. "And I was carrying around unwanted extra weight as a result." Nancy started out just by walking with her daughter. Then she started taking swing dance classes with her husband. "You get so much more out of life when you're always on the move! It's good for the whole family."

Hopefully, you're having a similar experience with your NEAT activities, enjoying all the fun there is to be had and lessons to be learned when you get up from your chair and see all that the world has to offer.

NEAT FUEL CELLS: Two-fuel-cell breakfast; two-fuel-cell lunch; two-fuel-cell dinner; one-fuel-cell snack; monitor alcohol intake

Many of my patients ask me if they need to take vitamins. If you are eating fresh fruits and vegetables with your meals as instructed, you're likely just fine without them. However, if there isn't a lot of variety in your diet, you could be missing out on some essentials, in which case a multivitamin will do you no harm and can provide useful health insurance. No need to buy any fancy, expensive supplements. Wal-Mart or Target brands will do just fine.

DAY 6 CHECKLIST: Today is a 6-point day

NEAT Feet: Three thirty-minute walks.
_____/_____/_____
One fifteen-minute walk. _____

NEAT Exercises: Twenty Core Chargers and eight Sunrise Stretches. _____
_____ points (2 points for the four walks;

331

0 points today for the exercises, but still do them!)

_____

_____

NEAT Beat: How did your planned NEAT activity go?
What would you do the same? Differently?

_____
_____
_____

_____ points (2 points)

_____

_____

NEAT Fuel Cells: Two-fuel-cell breakfast; two-fuel-cell
lunch; two-fuel-cell dinner; one-fuel-cell snack. _____
Number of alcoholic drinks I had today.

_____

_____ points (2 points: 1 for breakfast, lunch, dinner,
and snack; 1 for tallying up alcoholic drinks)

_____

_____

Grand total: _____ (out of 6 points)

_____

_____

Saturday is weigh-in day: Weigh

yourself in the morning and jot the number here. _____

Day 7: Sunday

NEAT FEET: Three thirty-minute walks and one fifteen-minute walk (one of your walks today should be outside, regardless of the weather); twenty Core Chargers and eight Sunrise Stretches shortly after waking

If you have been following the NEAT Plan, you have certainly lost weight by this point. Depending on how much you have to lose, you may or may not be satisfied with the numbers you're seeing on the scale, however. If you're feeling at all disappointed or discouraged, remind yourself of three critical points: One, there's a big difference between fat loss and weight loss. I routinely see clients who lose just a few pounds on the scale, but they've cut their body fat in half and replaced it with lean, toned muscle, which takes up less space but is heavier than fat. If you need to tighten your NEAT Belt and your clothes are fitting better, don't get too caught up in the numbers on the scale. Two, weight often comes off gradually in bits and spurts, just the way it comes on. Keep moving forward and it will continue falling away. Finally, the benefits of daily activity reach far, far beyond your belt size. When researchers from the University of South Carolina kept tabs on twenty-six hundred men and women age sixty and older for twelve years, they found that fit older men and women who were at normal weight, overweight, or even obese had lower death rates across the board than their unfit peers who weighed similar amounts. What's more, the death rates for those who were fit were generally *half* that of those who were unfit but weighed similar amounts. That means even if you're overweight, you are still reaping the life-extending benefits of a strong heart and much healthier body. It also means that being slim does not automatically mean you're healthy. You need to be active and fit as well.

NEAT BEAT: Pick up a puzzle

Today, I want you to seek out an activity that makes you think. It can be a board game, such as chess; a classic puzzle, such as a crossword or Sudoku; or a book of poetry. I personally love Dada poetry — you just snip words from a newspaper or magazine, place them in a cup, shake them up, and pull them out one by one to make a poem. An active mind is every bit as key to NEAT living as an active body. The brain is a large organ that requires oxygen and exercise, just like your heart and lungs. It also follows the same "use it or lose it" philosophy. By regularly engaging your mind and expanding your knowledge, you improve your problem-solving skills and boost your creativity. What's more, when you give your brain something to chew on, you're less likely to go hunting in the fridge to beat back boredom.

NEAT FUEL CELLS: Two-fuel-cell breakfast; two-fuel-cell lunch; two-fuel-cell dinner; one-fuel-cell snack; monitor alcohol intake; Cook-Something Sunday

Time to tally up your alcohol intake. Add up your drinks and divide the total by the amount of days you kept track. What was your average? For the best results on the NEAT Plan, I would like you to keep that number at less than a drink a day on average. Though one to two drinks per day is considered low risk, and maybe even healthy, you'll likely find that lesser amounts are more conducive to staying on track with your NEAT Feet, Beat, and Fuel Cell prescriptions. If you typically average two to three (or more) drinks per day, it is time to examine your drinking habits. Most patients I see who drink more than moderately do so because of dependency or emotional unrest. If you cannot cut back, please see your doctor.

DAY 7 CHECKLIST: Today is a 6-point day

NEAT Feet: Three thirty-minute walks.
_____/_____/_____

NEAT Exercises: Twenty Core Chargers and eight
Sunrise Stretches. _____
_____ points (3 points: 2 for the four walks;
1 for the NEAT exercises)

NEAT Beat: Today I performed the
following brain exercise:

_____

_____

_____ point (1 point)

NEAT Fuel Cells: Two-fuel-cell breakfast;
two-fuel-cell
lunch; two-fuel-cell dinner; one-fuel-cell
snack. _____
Cook-Something Sunday. _____
Average number of alcoholic drinks a day.

_____
_____ points (2 points: 1 for breakfast,
lunch, dinner, snack,

336

and tallying up alcoholic drinks; 1 for cooking something)

_____

_____

Grand total: _____ (out of 6 points)

Maximum points: 46
My points: _____

YOU HAVE MADE IT HALFWAY! Add up your NEAT points. If you've stayed on track and hit 137 (out of a possible 182), reward yourself accordingly!

11
WEEK 5: SELF-DISCOVERY

This week, you can say, "It's all about me," and mean it, because it is truly all about you. Now that you've passed the halfway point on your NEAT journey, it's time for some self-reflection: to look back at what you've accomplished, look forward to where you're heading, and keep in touch with the most important person on your mission — you! Some people are uncomfortable with this type of self-reflection, but it is a critical element of success.

This week we ramp up your NEAT Feet prescription, which will bring you to your feet 135 minutes per day. Remember, the idea is to keep your engine running all day long. Like your computer, your metabolism simply falls asleep when it's inactive for too long. With this level of NEAT activity, your metabolism will stay high and weight loss and maintenance will become much easier. Melinda, a thirtysomething accountant, put it this way: "I used to think I was active. Then I put on the Gruve device and saw that I sat the vast majority of the day. No wonder I couldn't budge my weight no matter what I did! I love the impact of getting on my feet throughout the day and doing little things. So far, I've been losing about a pound a week, but the best part is that once I get the weight off, I'll actually be able to maintain it. I've finally found something that works." This week's NEAT Beat prescriptions will focus on helping you establish the same positive NEAT patterns with equally positive results.

WEEKS 5 AND 6: NEAT PLAN COMMITMENT

For many, this is the hardest stretch. You may be losing steam, feeling the pull of your previously sedentary ways. You may feel like throwing in the towel. Don't do it. Once you push through this sticking point, you'll gain momentum that will see you through.

I am ready to commit two hours and fifteen minutes per day to my NEAT Plan.

I sign on to my NEAT Plan: _____

Day 1: Monday

NEAT FEET: NEAT Trifecta (three
forty-five-minute walks throughout the day);
thirty Core Chargers and ten Sunrise Stretches
(starting this week, split the exercises between
morning and evening doing half after waking
and half before going to bed)

You've arrived! This is the week where you start racking up the same number of NEAT minutes, 135, as our lean study volunteers. It adds up to three forty-five-minute walks per day, which sounds overwhelming, until you realize that every single time you get up out of your chair and move around, it counts. You can also divide the time however you see fit, so long as you are sure not to sit for more than two hours without getting up out of your chair. So, you can stroll on your treadmill for an hour in the morning while watching the news. Stand and pace while making calls for thirty minutes. Walk around the soccer field at your son's soccer game for forty-five minutes in the evening, and you've done it. You know what else you've done? Extended your life. Research shows that adults can gain two hours of life expectancy for each hour of activity, such as brisk walking, they perform. Let's say you do three hours of NEAT activity per day (including being on your feet for many of your NEAT Beats). You'll gain 91 days each year. Over twenty years, that's 1,825 days, a full five years of life. Even better, you'll still be sharp in your bonus years. A study by researchers at the University of Illinois found that three hours of activity a day actually *reverses* the brain shrinkage that is a generally accepted consequence of aging.

This week, I would like you to fill in the following sitting log for three days. Simply shade in on the time log when you sit today. As you enter the second half of the eight-week plan, this will give you a sense of your current peak sitting times.

NEAT BEAT: How do you define yourself?

In many ways, what you believe yourself to be is what you ultimately become. I'm not a betting man, but if I were, I would wager that your self-definition has either changed over the past four weeks, or is in the midst of undergoing a transformation. Today, I would like you to explore that further.

List eight words/phrases that describe you, starting with I am . . . (hardworking) or I am a . . . (piano player).

1. _____
2. _____
3. _____

4. _____

5. _____

6. _____

7. _____

8. _____

How many of those descriptive phrases involve NEAT? (For example, I am "active," or I am a golfer.) Now think about how that list has or has not changed from what it would have been four weeks ago before starting the plan. If you have not yet started to define yourself in active terms, it is time to start, because you really *are* active. The more you use those terms to describe yourself, the more they will become a part of, and partial to, who you are. And you'll start attracting even more like-minded NEAT people. Start redefining yourself today.

NEAT FUEL CELLS: Two-fuel-cell breakfast/lunch/dinner; one-fuel-cell snack

At this point, the fuel cell system should be second nature, as should the Eight Rules for NEAT Fueling (see pages 176–179). It will always remain, however, a work in progress. Take my client Mike, for instance. When he started the NEAT Plan, he became inspired to start playing in a hockey league twice a week. At well over 6 feet tall, and now very

A DAY IN YOUR LIFE (WEEKDAY)

Time	Activity	Sitting/ Inactive	Standing	Moving
5:00 a.m.				
5:30				
6:00				
6:30				
7:00				
7:30				
8:00				
8:30				

A DAY IN YOUR LIFE (WEEKDAY)

Time	Activity	Sitting/ Inactive	Standing	Moving
9:00	_____	_____	_____	_____
9:30	_____	_____	_____	_____
10:00	_____	_____	_____	_____
10:30	_____	_____	_____	_____
11:00	_____	_____	_____	_____
11:30	_____	_____	_____	_____
Noon	_____	_____	_____	_____
12:30 p.m.	_____	_____	_____	_____

A DAY IN YOUR LIFE (WEEKDAY)

Time	Activity	Sitting/Inactive	Standing	Moving
1:00				
1:30				
2:00				
2:30				
3:00				
3:30				
4:00				
4:30				

A DAY IN YOUR LIFE (WEEKDAY)

Time	Activity	Sitting/ Inactive	Standing	Moving
5:00				
5:30				
6:00				
6:30				
7:00				
7:30				
8:00				
8:30				

A DAY IN YOUR LIFE (WEEKDAY)

Time	Activity	Sitting/Inactive	Standing	Moving
9:00	_____	_____	_____	_____
9:30	_____	_____	_____	_____
10:00	_____	_____	_____	_____
10:30	_____	_____	_____	_____
11:00	_____	_____	_____	_____
11:30	_____	_____	_____	_____
Midnight				

active, there were not enough fruits and vegetables in all of the Midwest to sustain him. So we allotted an extra fuel cell for each hour of vigorous activity he performed. Problem solved. As you proceed, perform a similar self-examination. Have you taken up sporting activities that require more energy? If so, follow the one-fuel-cell per hour rule. Do you find yourself hungry at odd times of the day? Try rearranging your fuel cell timing. Remember move-earn-eat from chapter 5? As you change your movement patterns, the times of day you are most active, you also may need to change your eating patterns, the times you fuel and refuel.

DAY 1 CHECKLIST: Today is a 7-point day

NEAT Feet: NEAT Trifecta (135 minutes on your feet). _____

NEAT Exercises: Thirty Core Chargers and ten Sunrise Stretches. _____ _____ points (3 points for the trifecta)

NEAT Beat: Filled out How Do I Define Myself form. _____
Starting today, I will include "active" as

one of the first adjectives to describe myself. ____

____ points (2 points)

NEAT Fuel Cells: Two-fuel-cell breakfast; two-fuel-cell lunch;
two-fuel-cell dinner; one-fuel-cell snack.

____

____ points (2 points for all meals and snacks)

Grand total: ____ (out of 7 points)

Day 2: Tuesday

NEAT FEET: NEAT Trifecta; thirty Core Chargers and ten Sunrise Stretches,
half in the morning, half in the evening

Even when you're stuck at your desk, you don't have to be glued to your chair. Every half hour or so, stretch your spine and give your mind and body a break with this simple desk exercise. It'll help prevent that sluggish rigor mortis feeling you get from hunching over your desk and will keep your body from slipping into hibernation mode even if you can't leave your cube or office for a walking meeting or other NEAT activity.

Standing Twist: Get up and stand tall. Reach toward the ceiling with both arms, palms facing each other, keeping your shoulders down and relaxed. Take a deep breath. Then exhale while simultaneously twisting to the right and lowering and extending your arms out to the sides at shoulder height. Take another deep breath, bringing your body back to center and reaching overhead. Exhale and repeat to the opposite side. Repeat, alternating sides, ten to twelve times.

NEAT BEAT: Take your HAY score

HAY stands for "How Are You?" That's an important question to ask yourself every so often, especially when embarking on a life change, such as the NEAT Plan. Sometimes I find my clients get so carried away trying to please *me* they forget that ultimately this is all about *them.* So, while I am ecstatic that you're reading this book and following this plan, please keep in mind that everything you're doing, you're doing for yourself. My job is to give you the tools you need to get out of your mental and physical box and to live the life you imagine you can live. But it is your life, and yours alone. I want you to end each day thinking, "Wow, I did a lot today. Sometimes it was challenging, but I feel so great, it's all worth it," rather than thinking,

"Wow, I can't wait until this eight weeks is over so I can go back to living a normal life!" This IS your normal life now, so it's important to have a reasonably high HAY score.

On a scale of 1 to 10, with 1 being "I've rarely felt worse" to 10 being "I'm walking on sunshine," rank your general state of being. Circle the number that best describes your HAY score. Then, next to the score, write why you feel the way you do.

1._____

2. _____

3._____

4._____

5._____

6._____

7._____

8._____

9._____

10._____

If your HAY score is high, that's great. You are trending in the right direction. If it is low (below 7), write down three things you can do to improve it.

_____

_____

_____

How does NEAT figure into both your score and what you can do to improve it? For instance, if your HAY score is lower because you're struggling to get enough NEAT into your workday, it's time to reexamine your strategies. Maybe it's time to invest in that home treadmill so you can stroll while watching the morning news or enjoying your favorite prime-time programming. When you consider that the average American watches three hours of TV per day, you've got to figure that's the most seamless way to get ample amounts of NEAT without changing much else in your life. Remember, these changes are meant to be permanent, so they need to be ones you can live with . . . happily.

NEAT FUEL CELLS: Two-fuel-cell breakfast/ lunch/dinner; one-fuel-cell snack

Cooking is a great NEAT activity, but I realize that not everyone relishes chopping and sautéing and that there are those who would much prefer spending their NEAT activity outside of the kitchen. For these people, I recommend investing in a slow cooker, such as a Crock-Pot. These marvelous NEAT-living machines allow you to simply toss your ingredients (include copious amounts of vegetables) into the crock, and then leave it for six to eight hours while you go about your day. When you're done for the day, so is dinner. Since you usually make multiple servings in one batch, you're also outfitted with plenty of healthy leftovers for the week. Brilliant!

DAY 2 CHECKLIST: Today is a 7-point day

NEAT Feet: NEAT Trifecta (135 minutes on your feet). ____

NEAT Exercises: Thirty Core Chargers and ten Sunrise Stretches. ____
____ points (3 points for the trifecta)

NEAT Beat: My HAY score is ____.
My strategies for improving it are:

_____

_____

_____

____ points (2 points)

NEAT Fuel Cells: Two-fuel-cell breakfast; two-fuel-cell lunch; two-fuel-cell dinner; one-fuel-cell snack.

____

_____ points (2 points for all meals and snacks)

Grand total: _____ (out of 7 points)

Day 3: Wednesday

NEAT FEET: NEAT Trifecta; thirty Core Chargers and ten Sunrise Stretches, half in the morning, half in the evening

You know that NEAT is best spread throughout the day. Though that is preferable, I know it is not always possible. Here's what I don't want you to do. I don't want you to look at your prescription for three forty-five-minute NEAT Feets and not do any because you can't block off that amount of time at a stretch. It is *far* more important that you move whenever you can for as often as you can than to turn it into an all-or-nothing affair. For many of my clients, the workday is their greatest challenge. When it is simply impossible to hold a long walking meeting, take to your feet during the lunch hour, or walk and talk on your cell phone, then simply divide the forty-five-minute bout you would typically do midday into smaller, more manageable chunks, such as three fifteen-minute brainstorming breaks. Or extend the morning and evening NEAT Feets by fifteen minutes, and shorten the midday bout to thirty minutes. Then simply stand, stretch, and pace whenever possible during the day, so as not to go into hibernation mode.

NEAT BEAT: Design NEATercise equipment

Today, take a little time to contemplate a piece of NEAT exercise equipment you can build for yourself. Unless you're really mechanically inclined, this does not have to be the least bit complicated or fancy. For example, one man I counseled went to a hardware store and bought two huge bolts to which he attached nuts to fashion inexpensive hand weights for his desk, which he curled while talking on the phone. Meanwhile, Karen, a financial adviser, was inspired to construct her own home office treadmill desk.

"My husband bought three boards and a couple of brackets for about $40 at the hardware store," she told me. The results were brilliant. He fastened a board across the railings in front of the console to hold the keyboard. Then he hung a shelf off the wall where the treadmill faced to hold the computer screen and speakers. "It's not as slick as the commercial ones, but I'm excited!" Karen lost 40 pounds over the next six months!

Plan your NEATercise equipment. What

is it and what do you need to construct it? Where will you get the materials? Write it all down. Later this week, we'll put it together.

_____

_____

_____

_____

_____

_____

NEAT FUEL CELLS: Two-fuel-cell breakfast/ lunch/dinner; one-fuel-cell snack; Slow-Food Wednesday

Need more motivation to steer clear — way clear — of fast-food joints this Wednesday? Chew on this: Twenty-five percent of Americans eat fast food at least once a day, and one-quarter of all vegetables eaten in the United States are french fries. For the record, french fries do not count as your vegetable.

DAY 3 CHECKLIST: Today is an 8-point day

NEAT Feet: NEAT Trifecta (135 minutes on your feet). ____

NEAT Exercises: Thirty Core Chargers

and ten Sunrise Stretches. ____
____ points (3 points for the trifecta)

NEAT Beat: Designed NEATercise
equipment. ____
____ points (3 points)

NEAT Fuel Cells: Two-fuel-cell breakfast;
two-fuel-cell lunch;
two-fuel-cell dinner; one-fuel-cell snack.

____

Slow-Food Wednesday. ____
____ points (2 points: 1 for all meals and
snacks;
1 for no fast food)

Grand total: ____ (out of 8 points)

Day 4: Thursday

**NEAT FEET: NEAT Trifecta; thirty Core
Chargers and ten Sunrise Stretches, half in
the morning, half in the evening**

Did you get a good night's sleep last night?
A shocking number of Americans don't. In
recent years, the sleeping-pill industry has
been posting staggering sales increases. In
2006 alone, prescriptions were up by 15 per-

cent to 47.8 million and total sales of sleeping pills surged 29 percent to 3.6 billion, according to *BusinessWeek*. A culprit? Low NEAT.

Remember, your body is made to move, to expend energy throughout the day, every day. When you stay sedentary, you don't diffuse that energy, so it remains pent up, causing anxiety, restlessness, and — you guessed it — insomnia or poor sleep. Poor sleep, in turn, completely sabotages your metabolism. In a recent study at Stanford University, researchers found that body mass index (BMI) rose proportionately as nightly hours of sleep dipped below a healthy 7 1/2. In fact, the risk for obesity is 27 percent higher in those who get 5 to 6 hours of shut-eye a night compared to sleepers who turn in for the recommended 7 to 8 hours per night. Why? Because your appetite is regulated in part by two hormones, leptin and ghrelin, that work in harmony to help you maintain proper energy balance (i.e., eat enough and move enough). Those sleep scientists at Stanford also found that shortchanging sleep tilts the hormone balance in favor of ghrelin, which in turn triggers hunger and dampens your energy expenditure. Getting more NEAT will improve your sleep as well as your waistline.

NEAT BEAT: Use your mental energy wisely

We all think about ourselves a lot. And this week is all about you. There is one element of yourself I would like you not to think about, however — your weight. I know that seems counterintuitive. Don't you have to think about your weight if you want to lose weight? In a word, no. In fact, I find the opposite to be true. Here's a shocking observation I have made in my twenty years of practice: Most of my patients with weight problems think about their weight *at least five times* every waking hour. Imagine how much NEAT could be accomplished if that incredible time and mental energy were directed instead at thinking of fun ways to be active, such as creative cooking, or just getting up and doing some NEAT activity. Let's say someone worries about their weight about five minutes every hour. That is one hour in a day. Remember, every hour of just being on your feet, puttering about, is 150 calories burned. So simply being NEAT instead of worrying about your weight could help you shed 20 pounds in a year without doing anything else! NEAT living is about doing. It is about living your life differently. The weight loss is a by-product of that profound change.

If that's not enough to make you free your mind from weight worry, consider the science of "deflection" in problem solving. When faced with a seemingly insurmountable challenge, the brain actually works best when it is deflected from its focus. It's the classic "Eureka!" moment, where the answer comes to you when you're seemingly not thinking about it. We've all had those moments in the shower, walking down the street, or cooking dinner, but almost never when we're crouched over a computer trying to force our neurons into action. Weight loss works exactly the same way. It's natural to check your weight to see where your progress is heading; indeed, we do so each Saturday. But in between, cease to think about it. Simply continue living NEAT, and you will succeed.

If obsessing about your weight is a "favorite" pastime, list five things you can do instead for each time you think about your weight.

1._____

2._____

3._____

4._____

5._____

NEAT FUEL CELLS: Two-fuel-cell breakfast/ lunch/dinner; one-fuel-cell snack

Aim for at least one snack of crudités (a fancy French word for sliced or small whole vegetables) today. You can buy presliced peppers, carrots, and celery — even broccoli crowns — from most any grocery store. Many come with a little side of dip. Sixteen pieces of crudité equals about 2 cups of vegetables and has, if you go easy on the dip, very few calories.

DAY 4 CHECKLIST: Today is a 5-point day

NEAT Feet: NEAT Trifecta (135 minutes on your feet). _____

NEAT Exercises: Thirty Core Chargers and ten Sunrise Stretches. _____ _____ points (3 points for the trifecta)

NEAT Beat: I will not think about my weight, but rather redirect that mental time and energy to living a NEAT life. _____ _____ point (1 point)

NEAT Fuel Cells: Two-fuel-cell breakfast; two-fuel-cell lunch; two-fuel-cell dinner; one-fuel-cell snack. _____ _____ point (1 point for all meals and snacks)

Grand total: _____ (out of 5 points)

Day 5: Friday

NEAT FEET: NEAT Trifecta; thirty Core Chargers and ten Sunrise Stretches, half in the morning, half in the evening

If you work outside of the home, working more NEAT into your workplace is a must. Like most of my clients, you're likely trying to go it alone, brainstorming on the move, taking walking meetings with colleagues when you're able, and basically just getting up from your desk when you can. Today, I recommend that you try talking to your supervisor about making your office more NEAT for everyone. He or she may be more open to the idea than you imagine. The obesity epidemic is literally weighing heavily on our business leaders' minds, as sick days and low productivity cut into their bottom line. Health insurance companies are starting to offer decreased health insurance costs for businesses that offer incentives for their employees to be more active and healthy. Companies have started incentive programs that pay employees cash bonuses to lose weight. New NEAT-enhanced office buildings are springing up. In Silicon Valley, for example, I was involved in designing a building that was constructed around a central spiral staircase employees would use several times a day. Microsoft has built gyms within its complex.

Right here in Minnesota, I helped Salo, a midsized consulting company, install sixteen walking desk stations for eighteen of their employees to use periodically throughout the day. During the six-month study period, their productivity went up as their collective weight dropped by 156 pounds. On average, their body fat decreased from 31 to 26 percent, their triglycerides dropped from 143 to 73, and their total cholesterol went from a too-high 204 to a healthy 189. The notion of a static, boxed work environment is fading fast. Help your supervisor bring your department to the cutting edge by recommending some NEAT improvements everyone can do. It can be as simple as getting permission to hold brainstorming sessions outside, where employees will feel free to stroll around the office grounds while holding their meetings. Form walking groups at work. Or get his or her okay to use a portable stepper in your office or cube. If your supervisor feels included, he or she may be that much more willing to help for the health of the company.

NEAT BEAT: Improve your HAY score; plan NEAT activity for the weekend

Go back to Tuesday's NEAT Beat. Take one of the actions you listed to improve your HAY score. How easy was it? Did it work? Take a moment to explore the barriers that prevent you from taking these steps. If you're like my client Jo (and, in fact, many of many clients), I'm going to bet it's a case of too much thinking and too little doing. Jo made the classic modern mistake of confusing self-reflection with self-obsession. She didn't make a single move without thinking and rethinking and examining her past before moving forward. It's hardly her fault. The essence of modern psychotherapy is to look back before moving forward. Here's the problem with too much self-reflection — it *goes* nowhere. NEAT living takes the opposite perspective — move forward now, ponder along the way. Your HAY score will improve instantly once you take action.

If you haven't already, make sure you plan

a NEAT activity for the weekend. This week, since it's all about you, aim to do something you really love that speaks to the kind of person you are. If you're an introvert who longs for quiet time, plan a swim, a bike ride, a nature hike, or some other solitary activity. If you long for the buzz of people, attend a class you've always wanted to try or take your family to an amusement park.

NEAT FUEL CELLS: Two-fuel-cell breakfast/ lunch/dinner; one-fuel-cell snack; Fat-free Friday

Remember Fat-free Fridays include snacks, a minefield of fat in our society. Americans consume an astonishing 16 pounds of potato chips (that's chips, not potatoes) per capita every year. That's 38,912 calories worth — enough to pack on 11 pounds over the course of a year. You would have to walk about 130 extra hours to burn that off. Is it worth it?

DAY 5 CHECKLIST: Today is a 6-point day

NEAT Feet: NEAT Trifecta (135 minutes on your feet). ____

NEAT Exercises: Thirty Core Chargers and ten Sunrise Stretches. ____

_____ points (2 points for the trifecta)

_____

_____

NEAT Beat: I took one step to improve
my HAY score. _____
Jot a note about what it was.

_____

_____

_____

My NEAT activity for this weekend is:

_____

_____

_____

_____ points (2 points)

_____

_____

NEAT Fuel Cells: Two-fuel-cell breakfast;
two-fuel-cell lunch;
two-fuel-cell dinner; one-fuel-cell snack.

_____
Fat-free Friday. _____
_____ points (2 points: 1 for all meals and
snacks;
1 for going fat free)

_____

_____

Grand total: _____ (out of 6 points)

Day 6: Saturday

NEAT FEET: NEAT Trifecta; thirty Core Chargers and ten Sunrise Stretches, half in the morning, half in the evening

The key to successful NEAT living long term is being ready to jump when a NEAT door opens. How prepared are you to get up and go when a NEAT opportunity arises? It's important that you arrange your environment for easy spur-of-the-minute movement. For instance, do you know where your walking shoes are? Or do you need to hunt around for them every time you want to go out? Arrange a space in your home where you keep everything you need for NEAT activity — your shoes, keys, hat, sunglasses, backpack, notepad, pen, binoculars; whatever you need, be sure it's always in the same place, ready to go when you are.

NEAT BEAT: Craft your NEATercise equipment

Today, get the materials you need (if you haven't already) and craft your piece of NEATercise equipment. The purpose of this exercise is twofold. First it's to get you up and doing a creative NEAT activity, which is useful in and of itself. But it's also to get you thinking about what you need or want in your life to help you expend more NEAT. If you built a contraption with lots of exercise bands, that means you're looking for ways to improve your strength. Moving forward, you should include an activity such as calisthenics, tennis, or even simple weight lifting that will satisfy that need. Listen to what your NEAT device is telling you.

Note: If you planned a long NEAT activity for today, you can do this NEAT Beat tomorrow when you have more time.

NEAT FUEL CELLS: Two-fuel-cell breakfast/ lunch/dinner; one-fuel-cell snack

NEAT eating is not an all-or-nothing proposition. So often clients come to me and say, "I blew it. Yesterday, I had a terrible day, and I ate four slices of pizza and a pint of ice cream. I'm obviously not cut out for this." To that I say, "Nonsense!" Bad days happen to everyone. When one happens to you, shrug it off and just carry straight on. Do not look back. Do not analyze it. Do not hesitate. Absolutely do not blame yourself. Just move forward. You can make today a better day.

DAY 6 CHECKLIST: Today is a 7-point day

NEAT Feet: NEAT Trifecta (135 minutes on your feet). ____

NEAT Exercises: 30 Core Chargers and 10 Sunrise Stretches. _____

_____ points (2 points for the trifecta)

NEAT Beat: Today I made my piece of NEATercise equipment.
Jot a few words about it. What it is. How it works.
Where you'll use it.

_____

_____

_____ points (3 points)

_____

NEAT Fuel Cells: Two-fuel-cell breakfast; two-fuel-cell lunch;
two-fuel-cell dinner; one-fuel-cell snack.

_____

_____ points (2 points for all meals and snacks)

Grand total: _____ (out of 7 points)

Saturday is weigh-in day: Weigh yourself in the morning and jot the number here. _____

Day 7: Sunday

NEAT FEET: NEAT Trifecta; thirty Core Chargers and ten Sunrise Stretches, half in the morning, half in the evening

Be honest. Is your family helping or hurting your NEAT efforts? Sometimes those closest to us are actually those most intent on standing in our way. I had a client, Pat, who once started every sentence with "I was going to walk there, *but* . . . ," and each sentence would conclude with her not walking because her husband or friend or coworker was involved and wanted to drive or made her feel guilty for choosing to do something on her own instead of with that person. As we wrap up this week that is all about you, it is critical that you learn to stick up for yourself and, equally important, garner the support of others.

First, understand that change makes people nervous. When you make a profound life change, such as taking the NEAT journey, those around you are forced to look at their own sedentary lives. They may start to feel guilty or worry that you will now look upon them in a negative light. Your spouse and close friends may also feel left behind if you are embarking on NEAT without them. I encourage you to include your family and friends whenever possible. NEAT begets

NEAT. There are all kinds of ways to accomplish this. I have had parents put two treadmills side by side in the TV room so that dad and daughter can continue watching their favorite shows together. I know a mom and daughter who play music and dance in the kitchen for thirty minutes each evening while cooking dinner. I've seen parents play Dance Dance Revolution with their kids in the evening instead of vegging out in front of the TV. Each of these actions enhances rather than strains the relationships. If your friends or family won't join you, that is their decision. You are not under any obligation to stop your journey because they do not wish to take it with you. Just stand firm, explain that you are doing this for yourself, and, when possible, let them know your NEAT activities in advance, so they can plan around them.

NEAT BEAT: Perform your chosen NEAT activity

Also, look back over your NEAT logs from the week and get a sense of where you're still sitting for prolonged periods of time. Next week, see if you can target those periods, even if it means taking a simple stretch break.

NEAT FUEL CELLS: Two-fuel-cell breakfast/ lunch/dinner; one-fuel-cell snack; Cook-Something Sunday

If you have children, invite them to help you in the kitchen today and then sit down and enjoy the end product together. The family meal eaten around the table is the cornerstone of good nutrition, yet less than 10 percent of meals are eaten by a family sitting together at the kitchen or dining room table. More distressing: More than 80 percent of high school graduates in the United States cannot cook a meal. What possible chance is there that our children and grandchildren will be sharing family meals around a table if we don't pass down these skills? Remember, the best food is simple food. Roasted chicken and potatoes, a green salad, and a piece of fruit is an ideal meal that anyone can conjure up.

DAY 7 CHECKLIST: Today is a 6-point day

NEAT Feet: NEAT Trifecta (135 minutes on your feet). ____

NEAT Exercises: Thirty Core Chargers and ten Sunrise Stretches. ____ ____ points (2 points for the trifecta)

NEAT Beat: Performed my NEAT activity for the day. _____
Jot down a few words about where you went and
how you enjoyed it.

_____

_____

_____ points (2 points)

_____

_____

NEAT Fuel Cells: Two-fuel-cell breakfast;
two-fuel-cell lunch;
two-fuel-cell dinner; one-fuel-cell snack.
_____
Cook-Something Sunday. _____
_____ points (2 points: 1 for all meals and
snacks;
1 for cooking something)

_____

_____

Grand total: _____ (out of 6 points)

_____

END-OF-WEEK ADD-UP

Maximum points: 46
My points: _____

12
WEEK 6: KEEPING THE COMMITMENT

Twenty years of literature on weight loss, activity, and improved health can be summed up with one simple sentence: Greater commitment equals greater results. The NEAT Plan is a great commitment; but it should also be yielding great results, not just physically, but also in the vibrancy of your life. It's important, therefore, that you take steps right now, while you still have momentum, to ensure that you can stay on this path for the remaining three weeks and into the rest of your life. Despite what you may have heard (or perhaps experienced in the past), long-term weight loss and maintenance is 100 percent possible, if you take the right steps. In a survey of more than thirteen hundred men and women who had lost a substantial amount of weight, researchers with the National Center for Chronic Disease Prevention and Health Promotion found that after one year, two-thirds of the participants were either maintaining or still losing weight while only one-third had regained any weight. It's all about commitment to change.

This week's NEAT Beats focus on helping firm your commitment by making NEAT even easier to fit into your daily routine. Remember, anything that has you up on your feet and milling around counts toward your NEAT Feet activity. They are one and the same, not separate entities. Done together, they work wonders. "It's amazing that you can burn hundreds of calories just getting off your seat and moving around," said Jackie, a thirty-four-year-old mother of three kids under the age of eight, who shed 9 pounds that had been stuck for years. "There are so many opportunities to move once you're looking for them. My kids all go ice-skating and play hockey, and I used to feel stuck there sitting at the sidelines waiting for them to be done. Then I figured out that seven times around the rink is a mile. Now I get up and see how far I can walk while they skate."

Kenny, who cut his body fat nearly in half, has had a similar awakening. "I used to think exercise equipment was for 'exercise.' You used it when you were going to get changed into special clothes and work up a sweat. It's been eye-opening to realize that you can take all this great equipment, like treadmills and stationary bikes, and use them *while* you're doing other things. You can be productive *and* be moving." And that, of course, is the entire point.

Day 1: Monday

NEAT FEET: NEAT Trifecta; forty Core Chargers and twelve Sunrise Stretches

Are you still logging your NEAT activity time? As people progress through the plan, they sometimes start to slack off on tracking their activity because they figure they don't have to anymore. That's a mistake. Talk to any successful athlete and you'll see that he or she keeps daily activity logs day in, day out, year in, year out. Successful athletes don't really have to; but writing down their activity cements their commitment and boosts motivation (no one wants to see blank pages in their activity log). The thirty or forty seconds it takes to log your activity is well worth the lifelong benefits of more NEAT movement.

NEAT BEAT: Establish a Plan B

I have some clients who seem to live and breathe Murphy's Law: If something can go wrong to interfere with their NEAT plans, it will. So I impress upon you and them the importance of establishing a Plan B. Having a good backup plan means never having to say, "I was going to _____, but . . ." Ideally, your Plan B is something that can be done quickly and easily without leaving work or the house (which is usually the obstacle to Plan A). Here is a quick Plan B I recommend to my patients when they're unable to squeeze in their usual NEAT activity. It is considerably shorter than what they would typically do, so it isn't meant to be a substitute, but it is far better than nothing when their obstacles to activity are insurmountable. This routine will take less than ten minutes, can be done anywhere, and will increase your circulation, strengthen your muscles, and improve your mobility. If possible, follow it with a quick ten-minute walk.

Instant Pick-Me-Up

The Wall: Perform push-ups against the wall. Stand a few feet from a wall. Lean forward and place your hands on the wall so your hands are directly beneath your shoulders. Bend your elbows and lower your chest toward the wall until your elbows are bent at 90 degrees. Pause; then straighten your arms, pressing your body back to the starting position. Repeat twenty times.

The Taps: Stand a foot or two away from your chair with your back to the chair. Bend your knees and hips as though you were going to sit in the chair (you can extend your arms in front of you for balance). Stop just short of the chair seat and come back to a stand. Repeat ten times.

The Circles: Stand next to a wall and place the hand closest to the wall against it for balance. Keeping the outside leg extended, lift it straight out in front of your body, then circle it out to the side, around to the back, and finally to the starting position. Repeat five times; then switch directions. Repeat with the opposite leg.

The Extender: Sit in your chair with your back straight and abdominal muscles pulled in tight. Grasp the seat of the chair with your hands and extend your right leg, lifting it to hip height, keeping your right foot flexed. Sweep the leg a few inches out to the side; then bring it back in, and lower it back to the starting position. Repeat ten times. Switch legs.

Grasp: Sit in your chair with your back

straight and abdominal muscles pulled in tight. Place your water bottle between your knees. Squeeze the bottle for five seconds. Relax. Repeat ten times.

The Rolls: Sit in your chair with your back straight and abdominal muscles pulled in tight. Roll your shoulders forward toward your chest, then around and up toward your ears, and finally back, squeezing your shoulder blades together. Repeat five times; then switch directions.

The Dips: Bracing your chair against the wall or a stable fixture, grasp the chair seat on either side of your hips and scoot your hips off the chair, keeping your legs bent at 90 degrees. Bend your elbows and lower your torso toward the floor until elbows are bent about 90 degrees. Straighten arms and lift body back up. Repeat eight to ten times.

The Pull: Sit in your chair with your back straight. Take a deep breath. Then exhale fully, pulling your abdominal muscles tight as though trying to draw your navel to your spine. Hold two seconds. Release. Repeat twenty times.

The Squeeze: Sit in your chair with your

back straight and abdominal muscles pulled in tight. Squeeze your glutes (buttock muscles) as tight as possible. Hold two seconds. Release. Repeat twenty times.

NEAT FUEL CELLS: Two-fuel-cell breakfast/ lunch/dinner; one-fuel-cell snack

Just as you should continue recording your activity, it's even more essential to track your fuel intake. According to the National Weight Control Registry, which follows more than five thousand people who have lost more than 30 pounds and have maintained that loss for at least a year, one of the strongest predictors of successful, long-term weight loss is keeping track of what you eat. A prime example of the power of paying attention is Moira, a thirty-five-year-old new mom, who was *not* a client of mine, but worked with one. "I lost thirteen pounds through osmosis!" she told me. Which was funny, though not precisely true. When she saw her co-worker tracking her food intake, she decided she would, too. "It made all the difference in the world. Part of my job is meeting clients, which we do over breakfast, lunch, and dinner. And I always just let my eating happen. Now I control it. I look up the menu online and make a healthy choice before I get there. I record everything to keep me honest." The fuel cell system is designed to make tracking a snap. So keep it up!

DAY 1 CHECKLIST: Today is a 7-point day

NEAT Feet: NEAT Trifecta (2 hours, 15 minutes on your feet). _____

NEAT Exercises: Forty Core Chargers and twelve Sunrise Stretches. _____
_____ points (3 points: 2 for the trifecta; 1 for the exercises)

NEAT Beat: I established a Plan B for my NEAT activity today. _____
Write your plan down here:

_____

_____

_____

_____ points (2 points)

NEAT Fuel Cells: Two-fuel-cell breakfast; two-fuel-cell lunch; two-fuel-cell dinner; one-fuel-cell snack.
_____

_____ points (2 points for all meals and snacks)

Grand total: _____ (out of 7 points)

Day 2: Tuesday

NEAT FEET: NEAT Trifecta; forty Core Chargers and twelve Sunrise Stretches, half in the morning, half in the evening

My client Jason was despondent. Though he very much wanted to embrace the NEAT life and wanted to lose the extra weight he'd accumulated over the years, he couldn't fathom giving up his lifelong favorite pastime — video games. Jason was a self-defined "gamer" who spent the vast majority of his nonwork time plopped on the sofa moving little but his thumbs and forefingers as he slay villains and raced cars. To Jason, life without video games wasn't much life at all. Imagine his delight when I told him that even a gamer like himself could live the NEAT life. Thanks to Wii, an interactive gaming device that requires players to literally go through the motions of golfing, bowling, swinging, and kicking to play the games, Jason could keep his games and get his NEAT, too. Studies show interactive games like Wii burn about 108 percent more (about 100) calories an hour than traditional handheld games. In the end, he lost 40 pounds. Now that's NEAT living!

NEAT BEAT: Listen up

To truly commit to something, you must give yourself over to it 100 percent. That means using all your senses. The remaining NEAT Beats for this week will focus on making sure you are completely engaged in the NEAT life. We'll start with your ears. Hearing is a passive sense, but listening, really listening is an active process. Today, pick up your cordless or cell phone and call someone who would love a phone call from you (this is often your mom or dad!). Take twenty minutes to catch up on that person's life, being sure to really listen to him or her without allowing your mind to wander to what's for dinner or to an unsolved problem at work. As you chat with that person, and throughout the rest of the day, study how the words you and others use influence your general energy level. When someone compliments you by saying, "Hey good job!" or "You look great today!" it literally uplifts you, infusing you with a happy jolt of energy that you can harness for productivity and NEAT activity. What happens when someone criticizes you? You feel down, right? Gossip and harsh statements literally suck the energy out of you. You have more control over this dynamic than you think, and it starts with you. This week, make a point to use your words for good. Compliment people. Say positive things whenever you can. Notice how those around you respond in kind. Notice how it infuses the air with an energizing buzz. You can spread that feeling far and wide by picking up the phone and calling those friends and family members you've regretted losing touch with over the years. Start today.

NEAT FUEL CELLS: Two-fuel-cell breakfast/ lunch/dinner; one-fuel-cell snack

While you're working on listening, remember to pay attention to that little voice inside you that tells you when it's okay to stray from your NEAT eating plan and when it is not. There will be special occasions when, yes, NEAT eating will go out the window, and rightfully so. However, it is *essential* that you define a special occasion as something that is truly occasional, meaning it happens once a month or less, and is truly special. I have a client who suffers from what I call "special occasion syndrome." Specifically, everything from a distant coworker's birthday to a night out bowling with friends qualifies as a perfectly fine excuse to throw NEAT eating to the wind and indulge in a few slices of pepperoni pizza, an extra beer, and maybe some chips and cake, too. Each time, she insists that it's a "special occasion," when deep inside she knows it's neither, which is why she has unfortunately lost and regained the same 40 to 60 pounds throughout the years. Research finds that people who do not regularly cheat on their healthy eating plans are 150 percent more likely to maintain their weight loss than those who do.

DAY 2 CHECKLIST: Today is a 6-point day

NEAT Feet: NEAT Trifecta (2 hours, 15 minutes on your feet). ____

NEAT Exercises: Forty Core Chargers and
twelve Sunrise Stretches. ____
____ points (3 points: 2 for the trifecta; 1 for the exercises)

NEAT Beat: Called someone I've been meaning to call. ____
Used my words wisely. ____
Initials of who you called. ____
____ points (2 points)

NEAT Fuel Cells: Two-fuel-cell breakfast;
two-fuel-cell lunch;
two-fuel-cell dinner; one-fuel-cell snack.

_____

_____ point (1 point for all meals and
snacks)

Grand total: _____ (out of 6 points)

Day 3: Wednesday

NEAT FEET: NEAT Trifecta; forty Core
Chargers and twelve Sunrise Stretches, half
in the morning, half in the evening

Give yourself a pat on the back every time
you get out of your chair today. I've noticed
that people who tend to falter in their commitment to the NEAT Plan (and, indeed,
to any meaningful lifestyle change) tend to
be hard on themselves and beat themselves
down rather than build themselves up when
times are tough or they slip off track. On
the flip side, people who are positive and
optimistic, even during adversity, are more
successful at changing behaviors and losing
weight. Make a concerted effort to be less of
the former and more of the latter. It's as easy
as acknowledging and giving yourself credit
for every little effort. When you take the

stairs instead of the elevator, silently say to yourself, "That was good." Or "Okay! I did it." Repeat that positive mantra throughout the day when you stand for a stretch break, walk the long way to visit a coworker's cubicle, park in the far lot, and otherwise engage in all those little NEAT activities that add up to big results.

NEAT BEAT: Dress to impress . . . yourself!

Today's sense is vision, or, more specifically, what you see when you look in the mirror. How you dress is an expression of yourself. If you're in the habit of wearing formless clothes with little sense of style or pizzazz, it's not surprising if you end up feeling less vibrant or energetic than you could be. In Italy, they have a wonderful period every evening that is called, loosely translated, "the time to see and be seen." After work and before dinner (which is eaten very late in Italy), people freshen up from the day and set about walking and riding bikes around town. They wear casual but stylish clothes that allow them to move about while looking great. This week, make every day a day to see and be seen, even if you work at home or your full-time job is being a mother. Today and each morning this week, select clothes that make you look and feel good. Take care to trim your nails, fix your hair, shave, and take care of any and all grooming details. Notice the positive energy you feel when you look in the mirror compared to how you feel staring at a reflection draped in drab sweats or ill-fitting attire.

"But Dr. Levine, I don't have any clothes that make me look and feel nice." I've sadly heard that from more than one client. The task then is to pick up a magazine, such as *InStyle,* that covers fashion (but not something extreme, such as *Vogue,* that is meant to appeal to a narrow audience), and find some looks you think you might like to try. Then, this weekend, make it your NEAT activity to go to a department store and buy clothes that accomplish that look. You don't have to spend a lot of money. Going to Target or even the Salvation Army is fine. What is essential is that you make the commitment to yourself to look and feel great.

Also: No TV tonight. As part of "vision" day, you should devote the evening to looking at anything other than the television screen.

NEAT FUEL CELLS: Two-fuel-cell breakfast/ lunch/dinner; one-fuel-cell snack; Slow-Food Wednesday

Some of my clients swap their usual burgers and fries for deli sandwiches, like those from Subway, on their fast-food-free days. That's okay (though bringing your own homemade lunch is better), but realize that you still must make smart selections, and that chips and cookies still count. Sounds like common sense, but studies show that human nature often dictates otherwise. In a recent study, Cornell University researchers offered forty-six men and women a coupon for either a McDonald's Big Mac (600 calories) or a Subway 12-inch Italian sub with meat, cheese, and mayonnaise (900 calories). Those who received the Subway coupon were more likely to order a large, nondiet soda and a high-fat side, such as cookies, than those who went to McDonald's. In the end, the Subway diners put away a meal with a whopping 1,011 calories (five fuel cells!), while those eating at McDonald's ordered meals that averaged 648 calories (three fuel cells). When asked, the Subway diners also underestimated the calories of their meal by 21 percent. Read the nutrition labels and become an informed eater.

DAY 3 CHECKLIST: Today is a 6-point day

NEAT Feet: NEAT Trifecta (2 hours, 15 minutes on your feet). ____

NEAT Exercises: Forty Core Chargers and
twelve Sunrise Stretches. _____
_____ points (3 points for the trifecta and the exercises)

NEAT Beat: Today I dressed to impress _____.
If you couldn't find clothes to fit the bill, write down what you'll be looking for this weekend:

_____

_____

_____

_____ points (2 points)

NEAT Fuel Cells: Two-fuel-cell breakfast; two-fuel-cell lunch; two-fuel-cell dinner; one-fuel-cell snack. _____
Slow-Food Wednesday. _____
_____ point (1 point for all meals and snacks and avoiding fast food)

Grand total: _____ (out of 6 points)

Day 4: Thursday

NEAT FEET: NEAT Trifecta; forty Core Chargers and twelve Sunrise Stretches, half in the morning, half in the evening

Today's sense of the day is smell. You wouldn't think there is much of a connection between your nose and NEAT activity, but indeed there is. Just as a pungent odor such as the spray of a skunk can make it nearly impossible to walk without gagging, fresh stimulating odors can inspire and improve NEAT activity. Researchers from Wheeling Jesuit University reported that one such scent, peppermint, seems to be an all-purpose performance enhancer. In one study, athletes ran faster during treadmill tests after sniffing some peppermint than when they ran scent-free or sniffed other, less-energizing scents. Another reported that basketball players who inhaled peppermint odor enjoyed higher motivation, energy, speed, alertness, reaction time, confidence, and strength. On those days when you just can't get going, try splashing a dash of peppermint oil on your collar (at the very least, you'll smell good) or even popping a piece of peppermint gum in your mouth. The stimulating aroma works to lift your mood and may inspire you to move.

NEAT BEAT: Stop and smell the roses

My first love was Julie Jones. She lived in the north of England and I lived in London, at the other end of the country. Our relationship of five years predated e-mail and was based on handwritten letters. Whenever I opened one of her prized letters, the first thing I would perceive was the wonderful aroma. Julie would always spray her letters with a perfume she used. It was fresh and fruity with a hint of innocence. To this day, I am sometimes blindsided by a passing fragrance that immediately transports me back to that simple, wonderful time of life. Scent and memory are inextricably intertwined in the brain. The right scents can take you almost anywhere you want to go. Take some time to explore those scents that evoke positive memories that are happy, hopeful, vibrant, and alive. Seek out those aromas in the form of scented candles, essential oils, and fresh flowers. Infuse your office and/or home with your favorite aromas to create a positive mood that reminds you of your past and to live your present to its fullest.

NEAT FUEL CELLS: Two-fuel-cell breakfast/ lunch/dinner; one-fuel-cell snack

Imagine garlic simmering in olive oil, freshly baked bread, baked apples. Is your mouth watering yet? Tonight, wrap up your day of olfactory celebration by cooking up a meal that smells especially delicious. Take a moment to breathe in the wonderful aroma. Then bon appetite! Speaking of olive oil — another brilliant idea: Invest in an olive oil spritzer and use it to spray your salads and to coat your pan for sautéing. You'll save literally thousands of calories in a matter of weeks.

DAY 4 CHECKLIST: Today is a 6-point day

NEAT Feet: NEAT Trifecta (2 hours, 15 minutes on your feet). ____

NEAT Exercises: Forty Core Chargers and
twelve Sunrise Stretches. ____
____ points (3 points for the trifecta and the exercises)

NEAT Beat: My favorite scent (either present or past):

____ point (1 point)

NEAT Fuel Cells: Two-fuel-cell breakfast; two-fuel-cell lunch; two-fuel-cell dinner; one-fuel-cell snack.

____

____ points (2 points for all meals and snacks)

Grand total: ____ (out of 6 points)

Day 5: Friday

**NEAT FEET: NEAT Trifecta; forty Core Chargers and twelve Sunrise Stretches,
half in the morning, half in the evening**

Walk more, sneeze less. That's what I always say. A commitment to NEAT is a commitment to better health and well-being. Walking doesn't just help your heart and fend off big chronic diseases like diabetes and cancer. It also improves your day-to-day robustness by fighting off infections such as cold and flu. In a one-year study of 550 men and women, University of Massachusetts researchers found that those who walked every day had 25 percent fewer colds than those who didn't. Other studies have found that those who walk briskly most days a week are hit by half the number of colds as their sedentary peers. Why? Because your body is designed to function best in motion. When you walk, you boost your circulation, increasing the activity of the natural killer cells that destroy tumors and infectious agents in your body, and you beef up the activity of bacteria-gobbling macrophages in the bloodstream. The more often you walk, the more often you get a surge of activity in this important immune-cell army.

NEAT BEAT: A taste of something fresh and new

Today you are going to conjure up a new NEAT snack made only from fruits and vegetables. There are only three rules: It must contain three ingredients; it may include a dipping sauce, and the preparation/cooking time must be less than 10 minutes. Consider making fresh hummus (just blend chickpeas, garlic, and a squeeze of lemon juice in a blender) and carrots and celery. Use romaine lettuce leaves as "wraps" for a raisin carrot salad (simply mix shredded carrots and raisins with a little yogurt). Scoop out a cantaloupe and fill it with mixed berries. Use your imagination. The fresher, brighter, and more fragrant, the better. This should be a treat for all your senses, especially your taste buds!

NEAT FUEL CELLS: Two-fuel-cell breakfast/ lunch/dinner; one-fuel-cell snack; Fat-free Friday

Eat the snack you created today. This is actually a very important exercise, especially in today's world, where so much of our food not only doesn't resemble anything remotely found in nature, but also doesn't take a moment's thought or second of preparation. We just crack open the box or tear open the bag and dig in. This process requires you to think about food. What does it taste like? Is it sweet? Sour? Juicy? What flavors complement it? Can the food itself be used as a vessel? You're engaging your mind and literally consuming your mind's work. It doesn't get any more NEAT than that!

DAY 5 CHECKLIST: Today is a 7-point day

NEAT Feet: NEAT Trifecta (2 hours, 15 minutes on your feet). ____

NEAT Exercises: Forty Core Chargers and twelve Sunrise Stretches. ____
____ (3 points for the trifecta and the exercises)

NEAT Beat: I made a fresh new NEAT snack today. _____
Jot down a few words about what you made, what inspired it, and how it tasted.

_____

_____

_____ points (2 points)

_____

_____

NEAT Fuel Cells: Two-fuel-cell breakfast; two-fuel-cell lunch; two-fuel-cell dinner; one-fuel-cell snack. _____
Fat-free Friday. _____
_____ points (2 points: 1 for all meals and snacks; 1 for going fat-free)

_____

_____

Grand total: _____ (out of 7 points)

Day 6: Saturday

NEAT FEET: NEAT Trifecta; forty Core Chargers and twelve Sunrise Stretches,
half in the morning, half in the evening

For many people (like me), heat waves are as — if not more — challenging than cold snaps when it comes to walking outside, especially for those who don't like to sweat. Remember, your walks are not designed to be racing affairs. You do not have to truck down the street sweating bullets to get your NEAT activity. Take it easy and stroll in a way that's comfortable for the temperature at hand. Stay hydrated throughout the day and carry some water to drink and keep you cool. If you don't like carrying a water bottle when you walk, you can actually buy hydration fanny packs — belt packs that hold a small reservoir for water attached to a long flexible tube you can hook to your clothes for easy drinking access. As a bonus, these packs also give you a place to stash your keys, cash, and the like. Finally, proper layering is of the utmost importance. Many offices and homes have air-conditioning, so what is comfortable inside may leave you boiling like a lobster when you step outside. Wear a light-colored, lightweight fabric that will allow your body to breathe in the hot and perhaps humid air. And don't forget to wear sunscreen. It not only deflects some of the sun's rays, so you actually feel cooler, but it also, most important, protects your skin from sun damage.

NEAT BEAT: Get messy!

Remember what fun washing the car was when you were a kid? When we're young, we fully embrace the joy of digging into a messy task, such as giving the dog a bath. Today, rediscover the simple pleasures of a dirty job. Change into old clothes and clean out the attic, hose down the house, mulch the flower beds . . . the messier, the better. Get the whole family involved and have a blast.

NEAT FUEL CELLS: Two-fuel-cell breakfast/lunch/dinner; one-fuel-cell snack

If you ever watch a fine chef cook, you see that food preparation is a completely sensual experience. Even picking the right produce uses all five senses. You see the color of the ripe melon; pick it up and sniff it for fragrance; shake it by your ear to hear if its seeds are slightly loose; squeeze it to be sure it's firm, yet yielding; and then finally slice it open and give it a taste. How exquisite and wonderful a process it is! Contrast that with opening a package of Pop-Tarts. There is simply no comparison.

DAY 6 CHECKLIST: Today is a 7-point day

NEAT Feet: NEAT Trifecta (2 hours, 15 minutes on your feet). _____

NEAT Exercises: Forty Core Chargers and
twelve Sunrise Stretches. _____

_____points (3 points for the trifecta and the exercises)

NEAT Beat: Dug my hands into a dirty job today. _____
Jot a few notes on what it was:

_____

_____

_____ points (3 points)

NEAT Fuel Cells: Two-fuel-cell breakfast;
two-fuel-cell lunch;
two-fuel-cell dinner; one-fuel-cell snack.

_____

400

_____ point (1 point for all meals and snacks)

Grand total: _____ (out of 7 points)

Saturday is weigh-in day: Weigh yourself in the morning and jot the number here. _____

Day 7: Sunday

NEAT FEET: NEAT Trifecta; forty Core Chargers and twelve Sunrise Stretches, half in the morning, half in the evening

Once you engage in NEAT living completely, you set the stage for positive change of every kind. But don't take it from me. Take it from Dave, an occupational therapist. "When I first saw your research about the benefits of getting on a treadmill to read or accomplish work I dismissed it as an activity reserved for dreamers and risk takers. But I am a diabetic, a student in clinical research, and a father of two wonderful girls, ages nine and four. My health and concern for the future made me think there might be something to 'thinking outside the box' — or the cubicle, as the case may be. Now I walk on a treadmill while reading my academic materials, and it's changed my life. I not only enjoy working on the treadmill, but I've enjoyed many other benefits, including improved fitness, better-managed diabetes, finally achieving an ideal weight, more energy, diminished need for medications, and I can hope to see my girls graduate from college while I am living in an optimal state of health. Many thanks!"

Dave had ill health, a jam-packed work and study schedule, and plenty of reasons to throw in the towel. Instead, he took an opportunity to redefine himself and let a kernel of belief grow into a blossoming NEAT life.

NEAT BEAT: Believe in yourself

People often talk about having a sixth sense, like the ability to know something before it happens. I think we all have a sixth sense, as well — the sense of belief. You have to believe to fully commit to life change. Belief is like electricity. It is invisible, yet potent. It has the power to lift you from where you are ("here") and place you where you want to be ("there"). Without belief, there can be no dreams. Today, think about what you believe in and how you can reinforce your belief in yourself. Write down three things that inspire a sense of belief in you. Your choices can include religion, nature, even monetary success. Write whatever is truest to what really drives you in this life.

1._____
2._____
3._____

Now write down three personal qualities that help you believe in yourself (e.g., You're a hard worker.).

1._____
2._____
3._____

How can you use those things to reinforce your commitment to NEAT living? (For example, I have some patients who describe themselves as devout and for whom religious faith is a driving force. So they include prayers to help them along their NEAT journey. Others are outdoorsy and find belief in the power of nature. They include many natural settings in their NEAT journey.)

NEAT FUEL CELLS: Two-fuel-cell breakfast/ lunch/dinner; one-fuel-cell snack; Cook-Something Sunday

Have a lovely dinner with family or friends. Break bread together, and celebrate your belief in the NEAT life.

DAY 7 CHECKLIST: Today is a 7-point day

NEAT Feet: NEAT Trifecta (2 hours, 15 minutes on your feet). ____

NEAT Exercises: Forty Core Chargers and
twelve Sunrise Stretches. ____
____ points (3 points for the trifecta and the exercises)

NEAT Beat: Explored ways to further inspire belief in myself. ____
____ points (2 points)

NEAT Fuel Cells: Two-fuel-cell breakfast; two-fuel-cell lunch;
two-fuel-cell dinner; one-fuel-cell snack.
____
Cook-Something Sunday. ____
____ points (2 points: 1 point for all meals and snacks;
1 point for cooking something)

Grand total: ____ (out of 7 points)

END-OF-WEEK ADD-UP

Maximum points: 46
My points: _____

YOU HAVE HIT THE THREE-QUARTER MARK IN THE NEAT PLAN! Add up your NEAT points. If you've stayed on track, please reward yourself accordingly! (If you did not hit your point total, please reward yourself anyway. If you're still with the plan, you deserve a reward even if you've gone off course.)

NEAT VACATION

Everyone needs a break from their routine sometimes, even when that routine is the most perfectly healthy, natural way of life imaginable. Though I encourage you to take active NEAT vacations when possible, there will be times, perhaps once or twice a year, when you do not. Instead, you'll go to Mexico, sit on the beach all day, drink too many margaritas, and eat too many chiles rellenos. And that's a splendid thing. Those breaks should leave you refreshed and ready to return to your active life.

13
WEEK 7: YOUR WORLD

Interest in the "green" movement has soared in recent years as a growing number of people have become increasingly concerned about the state of our environment and the negative impact our energy-wasting lifestyle is having on the world. By embracing the NEAT life, you are doing your part not just to improve your own personal health, but also to improve the health of the planet.

Consider the simple act of walking. Meteorological scientists recently calculated that if all Americans age ten to seventy-four replaced just one half hour a day of driving with a half hour of walking, we could save 6.5 billion gallons of gas, cut 64 million tons of CO_2 greenhouse gas emissions, and lose 3 billion pounds of weight in a year. Talk about reducing your carbon footprint! All by simply using your feet. But that's not all. NEAT eating can have a profound, positive impact on the environment by emphasizing fresh fruits and vegetables and curtailing fast-food and drive-through dining. Our present enormous demand for fast food drives down the prices of beef and chicken so low that small, local farmers are forced out of business. Instead, we rely on factory farms and outsourced suppliers, such as Brazil, that pollute the environment. Fast food also uses tremendous amounts of packaging, which inevitably adds to the uncontrollable amount of garbage that is filling landfills faster than dumping sites can be found. By simply limiting the amount of fast food you eat and choosing to eat freshly prepared meals at home, you help increase the demand for fresh food, which in turn helps lower the price, which, as you've likely guessed, helps increase demand. As people eat fewer hamburgers, cattle rearing declines. And since each cow needs about 30 acres of grazing land, deforestation in Brazil slows. NEAT and green living are inextricably connected.

This week's NEAT Beats will emphasize your connection to your community and the world at large, helping you broaden your NEAT living circle. NEAT Feet prescriptions will remain largely the same, save a few surprises. And your fueling will continue to evolve, as we work on "front-loading" your day with fuel, so you have energy to burn all day and less to store at night.

WEEKS 7 AND 8:
NEAT PLAN COMMITMENT

Home stretch! By the end of these two weeks, you will be thinking about your time, activity, and life in a whole new way.

I am ready to commit two hours and fifteen minutes per day to my NEAT Plan.

I sign on to the final weeks of my NEAT Plan:

_____

Day 1: Monday

NEAT FEET: NEAT Trifecta; forty-four Core Chargers and sixteen Sunrise Stretches, half in the morning, half in the evening (note small bump in NEAT exercises; they will still take just two minutes to do)

Currently, 65 million Americans are overweight. The Centers for Disease Control and Prevention recently tallied up the cost of this crisis at $93 billion per year in health care. Though many think this astronomical expense is "someone else's" problem, it comes out of our own pockets, not only in health-care premiums, co-pay prices, and prescription drug expenses, but through our taxes. Every American citizen shells out $180 in taxes a year for obesity-related Medicare expenses. That's not even considering the price that businesses pay. According to the National Business Group on Health, American businesses lose $13 billion a year from obesity-related medical fees, decreased productivity, and absenteeism. Who makes up for those lost dollars? You do in the form of higher prices for consumer goods and services. We are all in this together. By taking care of our health through NEAT living, we ultimately improve our financial well-being and improve the general prosperity of our nation. Fiscal health, environmental health, and personal health are all connected. And you have the power to improve them.

NEAT BEAT: Locate your NEAT Network

As you learned earlier, there are quick-beat NEAT activators in this life, those people who get up and go even when life conspires to sentence them to the chair, and there are NEAT conservers, those who embrace every opportunity to take a seat. Given the sedentary nature of our society, it's important to seek out people who inspire activity, regardless of where you fall on the spectrum, but especially if you tend to be a NEAT conserver yourself. As you may have heard, obesity is "contagious." A paper published in the *New England Journal of Medicine* demonstrated that your social networks, the people with whom you interact frequently, even remotely via e-mail and phone calls, are key predictors of your body weight. If they are sedentary and overweight, chances are you will be, too. If they are lean and active, you will likely be as well.

Think about the people in your life. Who is a NEAT activator and who is a NEAT conserver? How can you tell? Those people who seem endlessly energetic and vibrant are certainly NEAT activators, as are those around you who inspire NEAT activity, like the coworker who's always looking for a partner to go to yoga class or take a walk at lunch. Those people who try to sabotage your NEAT activity ("C'mon, forget the walk; go to Pizza Palace with us!") are generally NEAT conservers, as are people who express contempt for activity, never walk anywhere they can drive, and move as little as possible. Your goal this week is to immerse yourself in a NEAT-activating network, spending as much time as possible with the activators in your life. Make a list of their names and seek them out. If you don't have many in your close circle of friends and colleagues, this might mean reaching out to those NEAT-activating acquaintances. Invite them for a walk or to join you at a gallery opening in town.

NEAT FUEL CELLS: Two-fuel-cell breakfast/lunch/dinner; one-fuel-cell snack

Just as our actions affect our environment, our environment's actions affect us — specifically, those actions taken by our government and the food industry. One such example is high fructose corn syrup (HFCS). Between 1970 and 1990, our per capita intake of this processed sweetener skyrocketed more than 1,000 percent, as the government subsidized its production and food manufacturers embraced it as a cheap, easy way to sweeten everything from soft drinks and ketchup to bread and salad dressing. The problem with HFCS is that our bodies may not process it as they do simple sugar. Though more scientific research is needed to know for sure, some studies suggest that HFCS may not prompt the production of hormones, such as insulin and leptin, that help regulate blood sugar and appetite, which in turn may promote weight gain.

Other research shows that drinks containing the syrup have high levels of reactive compounds that may trigger cell and tissue damage that leads to diabetes, which has risen to epidemic proportions in recent years. At the very least, it adds unnecessary sugar to many foods. When my patients ask me what and what not to eat, I tell them the simplest rule is "If you can't recognize it, don't eat it." That is, if you need a chemistry degree to decipher the ingredients on the label, it's not a very NEAT food. In my experience, the fewer ingredients there are on the label, the better it is for your health and waistline.

DAY 1 CHECKLIST: Today is a 7-point day

NEAT Feet: NEAT Trifecta (2 hours, 15 minutes on your feet). _____

NEAT Exercises: Forty-four Core Chargers and
sixteen Sunrise Stretches. _____
_____ points (3 points: 2 for the trifecta; 1 for the exercises)

NEAT Beat: Located my NEAT network.
_____

Write the initials of five NEAT activators you'll spend more time with:

_____

_____ points (2 points)

_____

NEAT Fuel Cells: Two-fuel-cell breakfast; two-fuel-cell lunch; two-fuel-cell dinner; one-fuel-cell snack.

_____

_____ points (2 points for all meals and snacks)

_____

Grand total: _____ (out of 7 points)

Day 2: Tuesday

NEAT FEET: NEAT Trifecta; forty-four Core Chargers and sixteen Sunrise Stretches, half in the morning, half in the evening

Our children are the future. The habits they learn today are those they will carry throughout the rest of their lives, so it's vital to engage them in the NEAT life as early as possible. One simple way is by walking to school. According to the Centers for Disease Control and Prevention, fewer than 15 percent of kids today walk or ride their bikes to school — a 66 percent drop from thirty years ago. One quarter of children get to school by bus, and over half get there by automobiles driven either by themselves or their parents. The government is actively trying to help change this through the Safe Routes to School program, which encourages such activities as the "Walking School Bus," in which a designated adult or group of adults "picks up and drops off" children at their homes (on foot) following a set route. This works brilliantly for people living within a 2-mile radius of school, as both children and adults can enjoy healthy, stimulating NEAT activity at the beginning and end of each day. If the school is too far away, you can choose a central location, such as a park, where parents can bring their kids and walk from there.

NEAT BEAT: Give of yourself

This weekend, you're going to volunteer or visit a volunteer agency as your NEAT activity. So now is the time to plan it. Do not panic! This should not be a complicated project. The agency can be anything from the local food bank to an elder care facility to a dog shelter. The activity can be taking a meal to a homebound relative, grabbing a plastic bag and picking up stray trash at the park, even just volunteering to babysit for a friend who needs a break. The most important thing is that the project is something in which you are interested. If you're seeking out an agency, research the names and numbers of a few facilities. Call them during one of your walks and find out their hours, what they need, and how you can be of some service. The activity can be as simple as dropping off gently used toys at a women and children's shelter or as involved as hammering nails for Habitat for Humanity. The NEAT life should be a shared experience. And no sharing is more valuable than reaching out to help another human being.

NEAT FUEL CELLS: Two-fuel-cell breakfast/ lunch/dinner; one-fuel-cell snack

Food is the potential energy for NEAT living. As I've suggested a few times, that means you should aim to "front-load" your day, so you take in more calories (energy) early in the day, when you have hours of activity ahead of you, and fewer later in the day, when you're winding down for a night's rest. This is extremely hard for many of my clients who are so accustomed to grabbing a quick bite (or, worse, nothing at all) in the morning, having a sandwich for lunch, and then devouring second and third helpings at dinner. Today, and for the rest of this week (and ideally the rest of your life), work on taking smaller evening meals. Plan your afternoon snack so it works as a buffer for your hunger and eat only as much food as you need to not feel hungry when you sit down for dinner. For me, this means having an apple or banana before I get in the car for my evening commute. You'll be surprised how little food it actually takes to feel satisfied when you take the edge off your hunger. I know usually food tastes good and that you'll naturally want more. The solution to that is to put down your utensils between each and every bite and eat far more slowly. This will allow you to savor and enjoy your food while also giving your brain time to get the signal that your hunger has been satisfied.

DAY 2 CHECKLIST: Today is a 7-point day

NEAT Feet: NEAT Trifecta (2 hours, 15 minutes on your feet). _____

NEAT Exercises: Forty-four Core Chargers and sixteen Sunrise Stretches. _____
_____ (3 points: 2 for the trifecta; 1 for the exercises)

NEAT Beat: My volunteer activity will be:

_____ points (2 points)

NEAT Fuel Cells: Two-fuel-cell breakfast; two-fuel-cell lunch; two-fuel-cell dinner; one-fuel-cell snack.

_____ points (2 points for all meals and snacks)

Grand total: _____ (out of 7 points)

Day 3: Wednesday

NEAT FEET: NEAT Trifecta; forty-four Core Chargers and sixteen Sunrise Stretches, half in the morning, half in the evening

At this point, you should be "addicted" to the buzz of NEAT. Human beings are pleasure seeking by nature. It is through NEAT that we explore our world, seek food and entertainment, find mates, and procreate. It is not at all surprising that we are not only born to move, but also born to love to move. Modern chair-based society has robbed us of that pleasure in recent years, leaving us searching for antidepressants, sleep aids, virtual reality, and drugs and alcohol to fill the void. By re-activating your NEAT instincts, you have effectively found a new "drug" to make you feel vibrant, happy, and alive. One of my most inspirational patients and a perfect example of NEAT addiction was Frank. When I first met him, he was a defeated man. Nearly a hundred pounds overweight, he felt like a prisoner in his own skin, confined to his car, cubicle, and evening easy chair. When I asked how I could help him, he said plainly: "I want my life back." I introduced him to the tenets of the NEAT life, encouraging him to start slow, first walking around the house, then the neighborhood, then beyond to the park with his two young boys. With each walk, he became more hooked, taking the NEAT mantra to his office, his marriage, and his kids. Two years later, he walked through my door 70 pounds lighter. "I played on the swings with my son today," he said with a giant smile. His dream life was just beginning.

Now that you're hooked, there is no limit to how far you can go to explore the planet and reach your dreams. Plan big. Think big. Use that NEAT energy to do great things for yourself, your family, and your community.

NEAT BEAT: Be heard; make a difference
The world is ruled by the laws of physics.

An object in motion (you) tends to stay in motion. And an object at rest (much of the world) tends to stay at rest . . . unless acted on by another force (you!). This is especially true of our political system. The status quo only changes when enough people pipe up and demand improvement. Today is your turn to be the squeaky wheel. Identify the world issue you view as most important and write to the governor, your representative in Congress, or your senator to let him or her know how you feel about this issue. If you don't know who your elected officials are or how to reach them, look them up at www.usa.gov, where you'll find all the resources you need to start affecting change. Remember, the politicians are working for *you*. You employ them and pay their salaries through your tax dollars. You have every right to tell them how you would like them to run your world. If you don't tell them the changes you want to see, they will never know — and the changes may never happen.

Also for today: Turn off the television for a no-TV evening and instead come up with a new exercise or activity to try Friday evening. Don't make it too complicated; a walk with someone new counts!

NEAT FUEL CELLS: Two-fuel-cell breakfast/lunch/dinner; one-fuel-cell snack; Slow-Food Wednesday

Need another reason to steer clear of the fast-food drive-through and keep up your NEAT activity? A Swedish research team recently discovered that those who rely on a steady diet of fast food and live sedentary lives not only gain weight, especially in the high-risk abdominal area, but also experience high levels of the liver enzyme alanine aminotransferase (ALT), which can be a sign of liver damage. Though the researchers couldn't tell which was worse, fatty fast food or idle living, it's clear that the combination is ill advised and most certainly not part of the NEAT Life.

DAY 3 CHECKLIST: Today is a 6-point day

NEAT Feet: NEAT Trifecta (2 hours, 15 minutes on your feet). _____

NEAT Exercises: Forty-four Core Chargers and sixteen Sunrise Stretches. _____ _____ points (3 points for the trifecta and the exercises)

NEAT Beat: I wrote to one of my elected representatives today. ____
____ point (1 point)

NEAT Fuel Cells: Two-fuel-cell breakfast; two-fuel-cell lunch;
two-fuel-cell dinner; one-fuel-cell snack.

____

Slow-Food Wednesday. ____
____ points (2 points: 1 for all meals and snacks;
1 for no fast food)

Grand total: ____ (out of 6 points)

Day 4: Thursday

NEAT FEET: NEAT Trifecta; forty-four Core Chargers and sixteen Sunrise Stretches, half in the morning, half in the evening

Reach out and NEAT someone. Are there hard-core NEAT conservers (read: steadfast couch potatoes) in your inner circle who you would like to move with a NEAT ripple? Instead of pushing them to do more than they might be able to handle, give them a NEAT nudge. Provide them with examples of how they can easily fit a little activity into their day and ask them to set an achievable target. Here are a few examples of other people's targets.

The mother of a sixteen-year-old girl with obesity and elevated blood sugar allowed the girl to talk as long as she liked on the phone with her friends so long as she was walking while she did it.

A sixty-seven-year-old obese retired gentleman committed to walking around the mall for ten minutes every morning before buying his coffee, then walking another ten minutes when he finished his cup.

A forty-three-year-old telecommunications executive purchased an inexpensive treadmill for her office and agreed to take all conference calls using a cordless phone walking at 1 mile per hour.

A forty-two-year-old truck driver agreed to walk fifteen minutes while waiting for his truck to be loaded, fifteen minutes on his lunch break, and fifteen minutes while his truck was unloaded.

A nineteen-year-old obese college student agreed to walk to class instead of taking the campus bus, accumulating forty minutes of walking per day.

A thirty-seven-year-old mother agreed to purchase an iPod for her son on the condition that he walk with it thirty minutes per day.

A forty-three-year-old overweight woman decided not to buy a plasma screen TV and instead purchased a treadmill for $500, which she placed in front of the existing TV. She walks at 1.4 miles per hour for the first half of *The Simpsons* (thirteen minutes) each day.

Each of these targets is well within the comfort zone of those aiming for them. The hope is that these NEAT nudges will put them in motion, so they catch the NEAT buzz, and keep on seeking more NEAT. Try it with someone you love.

NEAT BEAT: Share the wealth

Clutter is incompatible with NEAT living, as it creates a barrier between you and the items you need in order to get up and go. Today, sift through your closets and drawers. Pull out anything you have not worn in a year (special occasion garments such as suits and evening dresses don't count) and place it in a pile. Box or bag the clothes and take the bundles to the local Goodwill before Monday of next week. This simple act will not only open more space in your life to move and think freely, but it will enable someone less fortunate to enjoy what was merely taking up space in your life.

NEAT FUEL CELLS: Two-fuel-cell breakfast/ lunch/dinner; one-fuel-cell snack

It's true that unhealthy fast food is a growing export across the oceans and into the most far-fetched places abroad. But it's also true that we are importing rich, wonderful foods from those places, and our grocery aisles reflect broadening tastes that have been influenced by the cuisines of faraway lands. This week, seek out a food that is foreign to you. Try edamame, green soybeans popular in Japan, or adzuki beans, which form the basis of many fine dishes in India. Venture into the tropical-fruit bins for star fruit and persimmons. Try baba ghanoush (a hummuslike spread made from eggplant). Replace your potatoes with plantains (starchy banana-like fruits). You'll broaden your palate and free yourself from the food rut into which many of us fall.

DAY 4 CHECKLIST: Today is a 6-point day

NEAT Feet: NEAT Trifecta (2 hours, 15 minutes on your feet). ____

NEAT Exercises: Forty-four Core
Chargers and
sixteen Sunrise Stretches. ____
____ points (2 points for the trifecta and
the exercises)

NEAT Beat: Packed up unused clothing.

____

____ points (2 points)

NEAT Fuel Cells: Two-fuel-cell breakfast;
two-fuel-cell lunch;
two-fuel-cell dinner; one-fuel-cell snack.

____

____ points (2 points for all meals and
snacks)

Grand total: ____ (out of 6 points)

Day 5: Friday

**NEAT FEET: NEAT Trifecta; forty-four Core
Chargers and sixteen Sunrise Stretches, half in
the morning, half in the evening**

Throughout history, human beings have
invented machines to do work for them.
Ironically, it is we who are often the most efficient machines. Consider the combustion

engine. For every 100 pounds of fuel that a combustion engine burns, about 10 to 15 pounds of that fuel actually translates into mechanical energy; the rest is lost as waste. So the efficiency of the engine is about 10 to 15 percent. In comparison, the human body performs twice as well, delivering about 30 percent efficiency, or 30 pounds worth of useful work for every 100 pounds of fuel consumed. Think about that next time you're weighing whether to walk or drive anywhere that's just a mile or two away.

NEAT BEAT: Perform your new NEAT activity

Everyone, even the most active NEAT activators, fall into routines that threaten to become ruts. Ruts won't ever take you anywhere new, and can lead to boredom and sagging motivation. Every six to eight weeks, seek out a new NEAT activity to shake things up and potentially discover a new NEAT love. Some activities to consider:

Cooking classes
Cross-country skiing
Gardening
Horseback riding
Martial arts
Nordic walking (using trekking poles)

Painting
Pilates
Quilting
Softball
Strength training
Tai chi
Theater group
Volunteering
Woodworking

NEAT FUEL CELLS: Two-fuel-cell breakfast/ lunch/dinner; one-fuel-cell snack; Fat-free Friday

"I'm not hungry, but I want to eat!" When I push my clients to be frank about their eating habits versus their hunger pangs, that is the reply I often hear. They feel as though it is their weakness, but in truth it is their humanness. Homo sapiens have evolved to survive floods, famines, and natural disasters of every variety. It is deeply embedded in our DNA that if we see food we'd better eat it and lots of it, because who knows when we'll see it again. Your DNA does not know that you're living in a country where you can't walk into a meeting room without spotting a box of doughnuts or a cookie tray. How to cope? Trick yourself by chewing gum. Scottish researchers found that people who chewed gum after a meal reported feel-

427

ing fuller, had fewer food cravings, and ate about 40 fewer calories from sweets during the day than those who didn't chew gum. What's more, my own research found that gum chewing, which is a minor NEAT activity, can help you burn an additional 11 calories per hour.

DAY 5 CHECKLIST: Today is a 6-point day

NEAT Feet: NEAT Trifecta (2 hours, 15 minutes on your feet). _____

NEAT Exercises: Forty-four Core Chargers and sixteen Sunrise Stretches. _____

_____ points (2 points for the trifecta and the exercises)

NEAT Beat: Performed the following new NEAT activity:

_____

_____ points (2 points)

NEAT Fuel Cells: Two-fuel-cell breakfast; two-fuel-cell lunch;
two-fuel-cell dinner; one-fuel-cell snack.

_____

Fat-free Friday. _____

_____ points (2 points; 1 for all meals and snacks;
1 for going fat-free)

_____

_____

Grand total: _____ (out of 6 points)

_____

Day 6: Saturday

NEAT FEET: NEAT Trifecta; forty-four Core Chargers and sixteen Sunrise Stretches, half in the morning, half in the evening

Enjoy the beauty of the great outdoors today! As people commune more with their computers and less with nature, activities such as camping, fishing, and outdoor-based recreation are declining. Even our most majestic national parks, such as Yosemite and the Grand Canyon, have experienced precipitous 23 percent declines in visitors during the past twenty years. That doesn't bode well for preserving our forests and natural wonders. Nor does it bode well for our physical and mental well-being. People are meant to breathe fresh air. And it's certainly no accident that our skin is designed to turn sunshine into vitamin D, one of our most essential nutrients for life and good health. We are made to walk the earth. Make sure you do so today!

NEAT BEAT: Volunteer day

Perform the volunteer activity you planned for today. As you're helping others, keep in mind that you are also helping yourself. A recent review of twenty years of research on the benefits of volunteering found that this type of NEAT activity is tremendously good for your health. People who volunteer have lower death rates, less depression, and greater functional ability, especially as they get older, than those who do not give of themselves.

If your volunteer activity was short and sweet, perform your usual weekend NEAT activity. Otherwise, consider your NEAT Beat accomplished.

NEAT FUEL CELLS: Two-fuel-cell breakfast/lunch/dinner; one-fuel-cell snack

As you expand your worldview this week, experiment with new herbs and spices. Too many of my clients limit themselves to salt (which they usually don't need) and pepper (which is great, but there is so much more flavor to be had). Fill your shelves with cloves, oregano, coriander, cumin, rosemary, nutmeg, thyme, bay leaves, cinnamon, and basil. Or save money, buy some seeds, and grow your own potted-herb garden. Experiment with these flavors on bland foods such as eggs and bean dishes. These additions not only liven up your food, but also act as anti-oxidants and help fight diseases. Pakistani researchers found that just a 1/2 teaspoon of cinnamon per day could lower heart-damaging cholesterol by 13 percent and triglycerides by 23 percent. As a heart-healthy bonus, it also lowers blood sugar.

DAY 6 CHECKLIST: Today is a 7-point day

NEAT Feet: NEAT Trifecta (2 hours, 15 minutes on your feet). ____

NEAT Exercises: Forty-four Core Chargers and sixteen Sunrise Stretches. ____
____ points (2 points for the trifecta and the exercises)

NEAT Beat: Performed my volunteer activity today. ____
Note what you did.

____ points (4 points)

NEAT Fuel Cells: Two-fuel-cell breakfast; two-fuel-cell lunch;
two-fuel-cell dinner; one-fuel-cell snack.

_____

_____ point (1 point for all meals and snacks)

Grand total: _____ (out of 7 points)

Saturday is weigh-in day: Weigh yourself in the morning and jot the number here. _____

Day 7: Sunday

NEAT FEET: NEAT Trifecta; forty-four Core Chargers and sixteen Sunrise Stretches, half in the morning, half in the evening

Many of my clients lament being victims of their environment. Jay will tell you that you need to take charge of your world, especially when your world changes in ways that diminish your NEAT. Jay was a commodities trader on the floor in Chicago and then New York. "It was a very physical job. I stood all day, yelling, pushing, shoving, sometimes getting into scuffles with the other traders. I loved it. And I was always very skinny." Then he moved to Colorado — ironically one of the most recreationally active places in the country — where he sat planted in front of a computer from morning to night. He gained a lot of weight and felt achy and tired all the time. He tried swimming every morning for exercise. He gained five pounds. He considered dieting, but found it nearly impossible to restrict his calories enough to lose weight. "I knew the problem was sitting all day; it's just not natural." Inspired by NEAT research, Jay went online and bought the materials he needed to fashion a treadmill desk. He started trading while walking at just 1 mile per hour about six hours a day. After four months, he dropped his extra weight. "Now I have to eat more just to maintain my weight, which is a wonderful problem to have," he said. "I would never go back to a sit-down desk. It's not just the weight loss. I feel so much more alive and alert. I work better. I don't get sluggish after lunch. I have energy to burn all day long." Now that's making your world work for you.

NEAT BEAT: Start your own Buck-in-a-Cup Club

Get an old coffee cup and place it on your desk or in your kitchen. Every day, pop a buck in there. When it's full, put it in an envelope. When the envelope is full, give it to an organization that you fancy. It's a perfectly painless way to give more to those in need.

Also today, take a moment for some reflection. Did you give of yourself through your volunteer activities? Did you do your part to prevent hunger (your own) and excessive eating by front-loading your fuel intake and planning your meals and snacks in a way that kept you energized without leaving you famished by the end of the day? Think about your world and how you fit in it. Think about what you want from the world and how you can use NEAT to achieve your dreams. Get outside to commune with nature, energize your body, and calm your mind. This is your one life. This is the one world in which you have to live. Engage it to the fullest extent possible. Make it yours.

NEAT FUEL CELLS: Two-fuel-cell breakfast/ lunch/dinner; one-fuel-cell snack; Cook-Something Sunday

With an eye to the environment, many of my clients ask if they should be eating organic produce. Organic produce is becoming more mainstream, which is wonderful, as that means it's more widely available and less costly. So, by all means, "go organic" if you can find and afford it. The single most important goal, however, is to eat more fruits and vegetables. If buying regular, non-organic fruits and vegetables works best for you, do not give it a second thought. Buy that produce and enjoy!

DAY 7 CHECKLIST: Today is a 6-point day

NEAT Feet: NEAT Trifecta (2 hours, 15 minutes on your feet). _____

NEAT Exercises: Forty-four Core Chargers and sixteen Sunrise Stretches.
_____

_____ points (2 points for the trifecta and the exercises)

NEAT Beat: Started Buck-in-a-Cup Club.
_____

Reflected on my world. _____

_____ points (2 points)

NEAT Fuel Cells: Two-fuel-cell breakfast; two-fuel-cell lunch; two-fuel-cell dinner; one-fuel-cell snack.

_____

Cook-Something Sunday. ____
____ points (2 points; 1 for all meals and
snacks;
1 for cooking something)

_____

_____

Grand total: ____ (out of 6 points)

_____

END-OF-WEEK ADD-UP

Maximum points: 45
My points: _____

14
WEEK 8: GET STARTED

Your last week on the NEAT Plan is dedicated to *starting,* which may seem an odd theme for the final stretch. Why is getting started the theme of the final week? Because the idea behind the past two months has been to provide you with the tools you need for the NEAT life. You now have the knowledge. You have the cutting-edge research in health and weight management. You have learned how to set goals, how to plan, and how to put your plans in action. A NEAT life is one that is dynamic, healthy, and smart. A life where you fuel your body with the finest fuels and use your body to do remarkable things. Why would you put a time limit to such a great way of life? Once you flip the final page of this plan, you will not be finished; you'll have everything you need to get started.

This week, you will reflect upon the previous weeks to identify what NEAT tools worked best, what strategies you need to continue successfully moving forward, and the steps you've yet to take to reach those long-term NEAT goals. You will be equipped with all the tools you need. The challenge now is yours.

Day 1: Monday

NEAT FEET: NEAT Trifecta; forty-four Core Chargers and sixteen Sunrise Stretches, half in the morning, half in the evening

As you talk to your friends and family about NEAT, you likely feel a little ahead of the curve, since the science of inactivity and the need for NEAT are relatively new concepts to the general population, which has been so intently focused on purposeful exercise such as jogging and aerobics for so long. But I assure you that the NEAT wave is coming, and before long, it will be the word on everyone's lips. How do I know? The report from the President's Cancer Panel just hit my desk and — you guessed it — NEAT, walking workstations, and the need for less sedentary chair time and more natural human movement is featured as a potential strategy for beating back this terrible disease.

NEAT BEAT: Reflect, evaluate, and adjust

Your primary goal for this week is to plan your journey ahead. Look back through the past seven weeks and pay attention to when you were most successful and also when you were less so. What was the difference? This book is like one big toolbox for NEAT living. As with any toolbox, some tools you may find yourself using all the time; some not so often. What worked best? What didn't work so well? Are there still sedentary activities you haven't NEAT activated? Are there any tools in your NEAT toolbox that you haven't used? Write down the top three NEAT tools or strategies that you can make a part of your routine every day for the rest of your life.

1._____
2._____
3._____

NEAT FUEL CELLS: Two-fuel-cell breakfast/ lunch/dinner; one-fuel-cell snack

One strategy I like for both NEAT activity and eating is shopping the perimeter of the store first, and then working my way toward the center. This is great for two reasons. First, all the best stuff is in the outer aisles, because that's where the produce, fish, meats, eggs, fresh baked bread, and other natural, close-to-the-earth foods are found. Second, by the time you reach the center aisles, where you tend to find snacks, cookies, and sugary beverages, your cart will already be fairly full, you'll already have spent a good deal of time on your feet, and you'll be less tempted to toss all that boxed, processed food in your cart.

DAY 1 CHECKLIST: Today is a 6-point day

NEAT Feet: NEAT Trifecta (2 hours, 15 minutes on your feet). _____

NEAT Exercises: Forty-four Core Chargers and sixteen Sunrise Stretches. _____ _____ points (3 points: 2 for the trifecta; 1 for the exercises)

NEAT Beat: I reflected on what NEAT tools and strategies are most successful for me. _____ Which one will you use today?

_____ **points (2** points)

NEAT Fuel Cells: Two-fuel-cell breakfast/lunch/dinner; one-fuel-cell snack. _____

_____ point (1 point for all meals and snacks)

Grand total: _____ (out of 6 points)

Day 2: Tuesday

NEAT FEET: NEAT Trifecta; forty-four Core Chargers and sixteen Sunrise Stretches, half in the morning, half in the evening

If I had to name just one item that was iconic of the NEAT life, it would be the treadmill desk, because walking and productivity go hand in hand in human DNA. Since computers are only going to become more and more prevalent in the future, we had better find ways to move while we use them. The treadmill desks allow just that. "This has been a life changing event for me," says Terri, a forty-nine-year-old law-firm partner of her newly acquired treadmill desk. "I am about 10 pounds overweight and do yoga and pilates regularly. . . . However, I just can't find time to go to the gym. After work, I'm more interested in going home for a glass of wine than working out! In the first week alone, I walked almost 14 miles, burned around 480 calories a day, had more energy, drank more water, and worked more effectively. Thank you for inventing such an amazing thing (my

441

husband has dubbed it a 'tresk'). I have to confess that when I first learned about 'walking desks,' I thought it was the stupidest thing I'd ever heard. Then I visited a colleague who had them in their conference room. Over a period of two hours, I drank a Diet Coke, took notes, walked 2 miles, and felt terrific. I went straight back to my office and ordered one. Now I can't wait to get back to work on Mondays so I can walk again!"

If you can't get a treadmill desk for your personal workspace, it may be possible to convince your company to acquire one or two for common spaces, so workers can sign up to use one for one or two hours a day. A number of companies have done this successfully, and though sometimes the competition to get on a treadmill desk is "fierce," most of the time everyone gets a turn. And in the end, companies are often inspired to purchase more machines because it means a healthier, happier, more productive workforce. Better still, build your own.

NEAT BEAT: Einstein your home

Einstein said, "We build buildings and then we live in them." Meaning that our environment drives how we behave. Imagine a basement room with a great TV and surround sound and comfortable La-Z-Boy chairs. What do you think you'd do in such a room? Sit in front of the TV and eat pizza, of course! Now imagine a basement with a great TV and surround sound, but with two quiet treadmills perched side by side. What do you think you'd do in such a room? Walk and watch, of course. One of my clients set up her basement this way so she and her husband could watch the news each day and a movie each week together while getting their NEAT activity. Data suggests that the flood of sitting cues in our everyday environment is why many people sit all the time. Throughout the book, we've discussed ways to cue your environment for movement (including well-positioned treadmills). Now is the time to take it to the next level so you really do it for life. Go around your house this evening and in every room ask, "How can I NEATercise it?" It does not need to be pricey or complicated; just prominent. If you flood your house with these cues, you will have constant reminders to live NEAT-ly. Here are some ideas my patients have used.

- Exercise bike in front of the TV.
- Stretchy bands in the bathroom. Fasten the ends to sturdy fixtures and pull, row, and curl the bands while waiting for the bath to fill.

- Whiteboard in the kitchen on which you can list NEAT activities and NEAT tasks for the day and week.
- Yoga mat next to the bed. A reminder to move your body (i.e., Core Chargers and Sunrise Stretches) first thing and last thing in the day.
- Green fridge. Dedicate one prominent shelf in your fridge for only fruits and vegetables.
- Move the TV. One of the most successful strategies long term is moving your television from its prominent place in your living room to another room designated only for TV. By doing this, you must make a conscious choice to watch television, rather than just flicking it on and getting sucked in by whatever happens to be showing at that moment.

NEAT FUEL CELLS: Two-fuel-cell breakfast/ lunch/dinner; one-fuel-cell snack

Keep trying new foods. This is the key to not getting bored or falling back into bad habits. If you don't have time to learn how to cook a new food, simply swap an old standby with something similar, so the preparation remains the same, but the taste will be new, and the health benefits potentially higher. By swapping beef for buffalo, for instance, you get a better balance of omega-3 and omega-6 fatty acids and a leaner meat in general.

DAY 2 CHECKLIST: Today is a 7-point day

NEAT Feet: NEAT Trifecta (2 hours, 15 minutes on your feet). ____

NEAT Exercises: Forty-four Core Chargers and
sixteen Sunrise Stretches. ____
____ points (2 points for the trifecta and the exercises)

NEAT Beat: I NEAT-ened the rooms in my home. ____
How many rooms did you NEAT-en?

____
____ points (3 points)

NEAT Fuel Cells: Two-fuel-cell breakfast/lunch/dinner;
one-fuel-cell snack. ____
____ points (2 points for all meals and snacks)

Grand total: ____ (out of 7 points)

Day 3: Wednesday

NEAT FEET: NEAT Trifecta; forty-four Core Chargers and sixteen Sunrise Stretches, half in the morning, half in the evening

Don't underestimate the power of home decor (and I'm not just talking about treadmills in the TV room) to influence your NEAT activity. Research shows that open space (or lack thereof) and even the color of your walls can have an impact on how much you move. Aim to keep at least the main thruways in your house clutter-free so you can move often and easily. Add some red accents to jazz up the rooms you use most often. Red is a high-energy, stimulating color. British researchers even found that red-wearing Olympic athletes tend to win more often than those in blue (a calming color). Paint something red today.

NEAT BEAT: Identify your primary walking personality

What sort of walker are you? It's easy to identify by looking back and seeing what you did most often when you walked the most. Here are the most common classifications and what they mean for you.

Rambler: You love to walk outdoors. If that's the case, you need to plan your walks so you are sure to always be weather ready. I fall into this category, and I hate feeling cold, so I always have three pairs of gloves in my car!

iPod Walker: Plan to download new music or podcasts each week. Keep your player loaded and charged, so it's always ready to go.

Buddy Walker: Assemble a list of walking pals and schedule your walks ahead of time, so you always have someone waiting on you.

Shopper Walker: Protect your credit limit by going out most days of the week without your credit cards (or much cash). That way you'll have a grace period to think if you really, truly need that new tea set instead of making an on-the-fly impulse buy.

Chatter Walker: You love to chat and walk. You can do this on a ramble and/or with a buddy; but you can also do it on the treadmill at home. Remember not to set the treadmill too fast (no more than 2 miles per hour) and chat your way to good health.

Business Walker: Walk-and-talk meetings

are the ticket. In companies where this works best, people wear "Walking Meeting in Progress" badges so those around them know not to interrupt.

Daydream Walker: Walking is time to let your mind wander and be free. Walking may feel like a "guilty pleasure" for you, and that's okay! Just make sure you make time to indulge.

NEAT FUEL CELLS: Two-fuel-cell breakfast/ lunch/dinner; one-fuel-cell snack; Slow-Food Wednesday

As you reach the end of your official NEAT Plan, consider expanding those fast-food-free Wednesdays to most days. The scale will show it. A Temple University study recently reported that people tend to be about 1.5 pounds heavier for every fast-food meal they eat per week. Further, they found that people who ate fast-food meals three to six times per week weighed eight pounds more than those who skip the fatty quick fare eateries.

DAY 3 CHECKLIST: Today is a 6-point day

NEAT Feet: NEAT Trifecta (2 hours, 15 minutes on your feet). ____

NEAT Exercises: Forty-four Core Chargers and
sixteen Sunrise Stretches. ____
____ points (3 points: 2 points for the trifecta;
1 point for the exercises)

NEAT Beat: My primary walking
personality is _____.
____ point (1 point)

NEAT Fuel Cells: Two-fuel-cell breakfast/
lunch/dinner;
one-fuel-cell snack. ____
Slow-Food Wednesday. ____
____ points (2 points for all meals and
snacks and no fast food)

Grand total: ____ (out of 6 points)

Day 4: Thursday

NEAT FEET: NEAT Trifecta; forty-four Core Chargers and sixteen Sunrise Stretches, half in the morning, half in the evening

You'll notice that many of the people following the NEAT Plan talk about losing about a pound a week. Many are thrilled with that loss. Others, less so. If you fall in the latter camp, remember, you are building muscle through all your activity. That's a *very good* thing because it makes you stronger, raises your metabolism (so you burn more calories even at rest) and looks better, too. But the numbers on the scale move more slowly, which can be frustrating. This is why I always do body composition scans during our research studies. People forget all about the scale when they see they've lost 5 percent of their body fat. Pay attention to your clothes and your NEAT Belt; they're your best indicator of body-shape changes. Second, just as all those little NEAT actions can transform your life, that pound a week over time will transform your body. A 4- or 5-pound loss after a month may feel like a bit of a letdown. But when you're 50 or 60 pounds lighter this time next year, you'll be over the moon.

NEAT BEAT: What BEAT do you march to?

What are your very favorite ways to pass the time? Make a short list of activities you enjoy most with others and those you prefer when you're on your own. Going forward, the goal is to find ways to NEAT activate your favorite pastimes, especially if they tend to be NEAT conservative.

MY TOP FIVE WORLD ACTIVITIES TO DO WITH OTHERS
(e.g., sporting events, live music, museums, church events, dinner with friends, movies)

1. _____
2. _____
3. _____
4. _____
5. _____

MY TOP FIVE ME ACTIVITIES TO DO SOLO
(e.g., reading, playing music, surfing the Net, playing with the dog, gardening, shopping)

1. _____
2. _____
3. _____
4. _____
5. _____

Place a check mark by those that are NEAT activating. Write one way to infuse activity into those that are NEAT conserving. For example, if you love dinner with friends, simply add a walking activity, like bowling or window-shopping, before or after. If you love reading, consider doing so on a treadmill or stationary bike, or downloading a book to your iPod to take on a walk.

NEAT FUEL CELLS: Two-fuel-cell breakfast/ lunch/dinner; one-fuel-cell snack

Create a brand-new two-fuel-cell meal (can be breakfast, lunch, or dinner) today. You don't actually have to make it today. Just plan it out, so it's there in the back of your mind when you have a little time and are craving something different.

DAY 4 CHECKLIST: Today is a 6-point day

NEAT Feet: NEAT Trifecta (2 hours, 15 minutes on
your feet). ____

NEAT Exercises: Forty-four Core Chargers and
sixteen Sunrise Stretches. ____
____ (2 points for the trifecta and the exercises)

NEAT Beat: Identified my favorite pastimes and ways to

infuse them with NEAT. ____ Write down one that you will do this weekend.

_____

____ **points (2** points)

_____

_____

NEAT Fuel Cells: Two-fuel-cell breakfast/ lunch/dinner; one-fuel-cell snack. ____ ____ points (2 points for all meals and snacks)

_____

_____

Grand total: ____ (out of 6 points)

_____

Day 5: Friday

NEAT FEET: NEAT Trifecta; forty-four Core Chargers and sixteen Sunrise Stretches, half in the morning, half in the afternoon

How are your shoes holding up? Your primary walking shoes should be replaced every 300 to 500 miles (or every three to six months), depending on how sturdy they are; how hard you are on them; and the type of surfaces on which you walk (cement being the hardest; soft paths the easiest). Walking in worn-out shoes can lead to nagging aches and pains during and after your walks. If you've been following the plan faithfully, you'll be due to replace yours soon. Mark a date on the calendar not further out than four more weeks and treat yourself to a new pair.

NEAT BEAT: Check in

Remember your plant? (For its sake I hope you do.) How much has it grown over the past seven weeks? Does it look healthy and well tended? Or has it withered from being neglected? It is a symbol of your NEAT life, vibrant, ever growing, making your world a healthier place. Remember to care for it and yourself. Which means taking your HAY ("How Are You?") score again.

On a scale of 1 to 10, with 1 being "I've rarely felt worse" to 10 being "I'm walking on sunshine," rank your general state of being. Circle the number that best describes your HAY score. Then, next to the score, write a few notes regarding why you feel the way you do.

1._____
2._____
3._____
4._____
5._____
6._____
7._____
8._____

9._____

10._____

How does this compare to your HAY score from 3 weeks ago?

_____

_____

If your HAY score is higher, that's great. You are trending in the right direction. If it is lower, write down three things you can do to improve it, and start one of them now.

1._____

2._____

3._____

NEAT FUEL CELLS: Two-fuel-cell breakfast/ lunch/dinner; one-fuel-cell snack; Fat-free Friday

If you aren't currently having some citrus fruit every day, consider starting now and making it a daily habit. Vitamin C, a prominent nutrient in citrus fruits, has been found to improve the health of your cartilage (important for healthy knees!), prevent heart disease, lower cancer risk, and even prevent wrinkles. All that from a little orange! My personal favorite are clementines — so sweet, portable, and easy to peel without making a mess.

DAY 5 CHECKLIST: Today is a 7-point day

NEAT Feet: NEAT Trifecta (2 hours, 15 minutes on your feet). ____

NEAT Exercises: Forty-four Core Chargers and
sixteen Sunrise Stretches. ____
____ points (2 points for the trifecta and the exercises)

NEAT Beat: I checked in on my plant. It is now ____ inches tall.
I checked my HAY score. It is higher ____ lower ____ same ____.
____ points (3 points)

NEAT Fuel Cells: Two-fuel-cell breakfast/ lunch/dinner;
one-fuel-cell snack. ____
Fat-free Friday. ____
____ points (2 points: 1 for all meals and snacks;
1 for going fat-free)

Day 6: Saturday

NEAT FEET: NEAT Trifecta; forty-four Core Chargers and sixteen Sunrise Stretches, half in the morning, half in the evening

"Can I walk with weights?" my clients often ask, eager to coax more progress from each NEAT step. The simple answer is no. Carrying weights on a walk doesn't provide the right resistance to tone your muscles. And though it may increase your calorie burn slightly by making your walking harder and raising your heart rate, those slight gains are not worth the risks. Carrying weights strains your shoulder and elbow ligaments and tendons and can cause joint problems, and can increase your blood pressure in unhealthy ways. Better to drop the weights and pick up the pace if you're looking for greater gains.

NEAT BEAT: Where are you on the road to your NEAT Goals?

How far along are you in meeting your NEAT Goals (see page 132)? Which ones have you met? Which ones have fallen by the wayside? It's time to revisit them and make sure that you stay on the path to those goals and dreams that are most important to you. Today, write down the next five steps to your most important goal. (If you've already met your most important goal, bravo! Write down the steps to the next one on the list.)

1._____
2._____
3._____
4._____
5._____

NEAT FUEL CELLS: Two-fuel-cell breakfast/ lunch/dinner; one-fuel-cell snack

Eating organic may not always be necessary, but one green grocery habit you should definitely adopt is reusable shopping bags. Americans go through 100 billion plastic shopping bags each year and recycle fewer than 1 percent of them. Some stores in California have started banning these environmental bombs. Unless you recycle them or put them to good use in your household, I suggest you do the same. Most grocery stores now sell cloth totes you can purchase for $1 (which, incidentally hold more, are easier to carry, and don't tear through). Stock up next time you shop.

DAY 6 CHECKLIST: Today is a 7-point day

NEAT Feet: NEAT Trifecta (2 hours, 15 minutes on your feet). _____

NEAT Exercises: Forty-four Core Chargers and
sixteen Sunrise Stretches. _____
_____ points (2 points for the trifecta and the exercises)

NEAT Beat: I have assessed my progress toward my NEAT goals. _____.
Write down the one step you will take today to
move closer to them.

_____ points (4 points)

NEAT Fuel Cells: Two-fuel-cell breakfast/ lunch/dinner;
one-fuel-cell snack. _____
_____ point (1 point for all meals and snacks)

Grand total: _____ (out of 7 points)

459

Day 7: Sunday

NEAT FEET: NEAT Trifecta; forty-four Core Chargers and sixteen Sunrise Stretches, half in the morning, half in the evening

Wake up early and take a fabulous walk today. Give thanks for the people in your life; for the work that you do; for the ability to use your mind, spirit, and feet to carry you into a better way of life. You become those things that you repeatedly do every day. Make NEAT priority one. It will positively affect everything else, just like the tenets of NEAT living.

NEAT BEAT: Party!

Celebrate today. Invite friends to go bowling. Go fly kites and have a picnic in the park. Go skiing for the day. Go to the beach. You have accomplished great changes these past two months. Embrace today in the most enjoyable NEAT way possible.

NEAT FUEL CELLS: Two-fuel-cell breakfast/ lunch/dinner; one-fuel-cell snack; Cook-Something Sunday

460

Continue the celebratory theme into dinnertime by cooking up something special tonight. Go ahead and bake something decadent. There's no harm in the occasional sweet when you're living an active life on your feet. Invite your friends and family to share your meal and toast the beginning of the rest of your NEAT life.

DAY 7 CHECKLIST: Today is a 7-point day

NEAT Feet: NEAT Trifecta (2 hours, 15 minutes on your feet). ____

NEAT Exercises: Forty-four Core Chargers and sixteen Sunrise Stretches. ____

____ points (3 points for the trifecta and the exercises)

NEAT Beat: Celebrate! Write a few words about your NEAT party.

____ points (2 points)

461

NEAT Fuel Cells: Two-fuel-cell breakfast/
lunch/dinner;
one-fuel-cell snack. ____
Cook-Something Sunday. ____
____ (2 points: 1 for all meals and snacks;
1 for cooking something)

Grand total: ____ (out of 7 points)

END-OF-WEEK ADD-UP

Maximum points: 46
My points: _____

YOU HAVE DONE IT! Add up your NEAT points. The grand total is 365, one for every day of the year, which you are now going to live vibrantly and actively. If you've stayed on track and reached 275 points (75 percent of 365), please reward yourself accordingly. Even if you fell short of that mark, please do reward yourself with something. In the long run, it does not matter if you did not do everything; that was not the intent. The point was to examine and try a completely new way of living. You have now started a NEAT life. Enjoy the day. Well done. Cheers!

■ ■ ■ ■

PART 3
THE FUTURE

■ ■ ■ ■

15
THE NEAT FUTURE
IT'S COMING, AND YOU'RE LEADING THE WAY

We are standing on the edge of a NEAT wave. You and I, and all the early adopters of the NEAT life may be the first to hop aboard, but you will soon look back and see millions of people joining along.

NEAT is the undeniable future. The health-care system is currently burdened with shelling out $117 billion a year for overweight-related health problems. It's a price tag we as health-care premium payers can no longer afford. Even the government now recognizes NEAT is the answer. The Centers for Disease Control recently conducted a study that estimated that if the 88 million sedentary people in this country got more moderate (read "NEAT") activity, we could reduce yearly medical costs by as much as $76.6 billion.

Employers are starting to pay attention, too. Workplace physical activity programs have been shown to reduce sick days by up to 32 percent, slash corporate health-care costs by up to 55 percent, and increase productivity by 52 percent. I've seen those exact benefits in every workplace study I've done. Instead of nodding off from 2 p.m. to 4 p.m., employees are literally buzzing with energy. People feel better, think more clearly, and catch fewer colds. Regular activity lowers the risk of almost every disease known to man, including heart disease, diabetes, cancer, osteoporosis, Alzheimer's, and depression. Those diseases take their toll on us financially as well as physically and emotionally. We simply cannot afford to continue down this chair-centric existence. You know it. I know it. The rest of the world is coming to know it, too.

THE NEAT MOVEMENT MARCHES ON

In many ways, the NEAT movement is an unstoppable force, paramount to creating a sustainable, healthy future for us and our children. Increasingly, you see homes, offices, and communities being engineered to encourage more NEAT activity.

Major cities such as London and New York City are charging congestion taxes on cars that drive into their midtown areas with the purpose of getting more people off the street and on their feet. The U.S. government is calling for the public and private sectors to work together to make it easier and more enjoyable for people to live more active lives. It is currently crafting the Physical Activities Guidelines for Americans Act, which will promote better physical activity guidelines for all Americans. "The wealthiest country in the world should be the healthiest. This is a matter of national security and of economic competitiveness," said Congressman Mark Udall (Colorado). "These guidelines are a commonsense way to improve the quality of life of many Americans." Congressman Zach Wamp (Tennessee) echoed these sentiments: "The human body was made to move."

Towns across the nation are passing ordinances demanding sidewalks so residents can safely walk from their homes to the downtown, which in many cases are just a few short blocks away. You'll soon see NEAT workplaces buzzing with treadmill desks and NEAT cities and towns complete with networks of pedestrian pathways. NEAT will even take center stage in our homes and schools.

The New York Times Magazine recently ran a marvelous piece titled "Eco-House for the Future." In it, the architectural visionaries at Diller Scofidio + Renfro dreamed up a "guilt-free, sustainable luxury house that thrives on excess." Notably, it contains a "WorkOut Generator," a treadmill with a hands-free headset the homeowner can use to talk and walk, which also converts the energy expended on the treadmill into a 110-volt AC, which in turn feeds a storage battery in the house; a "DryerCloset," a contraption that automatically shuttles hung clothes back and forth from open-air spaces in the house, so residents can line dry their clothes with ease; and a "PiezoSleeper" that incorporates transducers in the mattress to collect and convert excess human energy into electricity, which is stored in the house's rechargeable battery. At a recent National Ergonomics Conference, a whole afternoon was devoted to NEAT homes, NEAT workplaces, NEAT retirement homes, and NEAT schools. I recently learned that some supermarkets in England are offering shoppers a "trim trolley," a shopping cart that helps people burn more calories while they shop. Increase the resistance of the cart and a person can burn about 280 calories while pushing it up and down the aisles during a forty-minute shopping trip. How positively NEAT!

Forward-thinking scientists are also at work on our nation's schools. My team designed an entire 55,000-square-foot NEAT school space we called "the Neighborhood," which resembled a village square. The actual "classroom" was a plasticized hockey rink complete with standing desks and vertical, mobile whiteboards that allowed for activity-permissive lessons. The Neighborhood also included miniature golf, basketball hoops, indoor soccer, climbing mazes, and activity-promoting games. The children used wireless laptop computers and portable video display units to facilitate mobile learning. Children were allowed to move throughout the Neighborhood during lesson plans. The entire space allowed kids to do what they very naturally do — *move.* Did their academics suffer? Quite the contrary. They performed just as well and were happier and more engaged. More telling, they even asked if they could come *back to school* in the evenings to do their homework. School was now a cool place to be! The kids are our future, and they love NEAT.

More remarkable are the people I meet every day who are deciding that they've had enough of being a slave to their cars and chained to their chairs and are taking action to live more full, active, fulfilling lives. I've seen clients take up dancing, singing, ice-skating, hockey, and bowling. I've seen them remodel their homes, create lush, beautiful gardens, and go on active vacations. I can see the transformative power of even the smallest NEAT action, like turning off the TV for an hour and going for a walk. That is the true power of the NEAT movement — taking control of your life.

JUST DO IT

The bottom line is that human beings are a species of doers, and NEAT is all about doing. We've engineered ourselves into these chairs, and we're going to rise up and find our way back out of them. The world is moving in that direction, but, in the meantime, it starts with *you* and the way *you* live *your* life.

The bottom line of the NEAT life is DO. Many of my clients come in feeling trapped by their weight and burdened by life. They want to do something special with their lives, but feel they cannot because they are stuck and don't know how to begin freeing themselves. What you've learned and practiced in the pages of this book is the first (and next and every other) step. It's about shaking off the past and deciding to live differently. The choice is all yours. You can choose to spend your life in the observer's chair, or you can choose to get up and join the game. You can choose to sit and watch the Travel Channel, or you can get up and explore our beautiful world. You can choose to sit entrapped by the computer stream of e-mail, or you can get up and talk with your colleague as you walk. You can choose to sit at home and watch your child unwrap his first insulin syringe, or you can get up and take him to the park. You can choose to sit by and watch your life go by, or you can get up and live it.

The great mistake I see people make time and time again is to look at all the steps they need to take to reach their goals, whether they be weight or otherwise, and become too paralyzed to take even one. Don't be. Life isn't just a journey. It's your journey. Sure, you can stop and park yourself in the same place for five or ten years. Or you can get up and put one foot in front of the other every day as you make your way toward your dreams. Time passes either way. But by taking the latter, NEAT approach, you can actually get to all those places you dream about reaching in your life.

Take Gina, a single mother of two young children, for example. She worked in the filing department at a company I was visiting in California. She started asking me questions about how to lose weight, but I sensed her dissatisfaction wasn't really about her dress size. So I asked what she really wanted to do in life. She said, "I've always wanted to go to law school. But I never even graduated high school." I mentioned that the local high school has a program to help people get their GRE and that they might even have day care. That was the end of our conversation . . . until about five years later. I received a handwritten letter from a law firm. It was from Gina. She had lost the weight. But that's not really what she wanted to tell me. The big news was that she had gotten her GRE, then found a program through the University of California that helped single moms attend college. From the letterhead, I could see that she was now chief paralegal of a law firm. Even better, attached to the note was her acceptance letter to the UCLA School of Law. Gina had done it. She had taken the steps and was on the path to her dreams.

That is what I want for you. Yes, the NEAT life will establish the NEAT activity and food habits that enable you to shed pounds and be healthier. But I want far, far more for you than that. I want you to be true to yourself. I want you to stand before the mirror and say what it is you want from your body, your mind, your soul, and your

NEAT. Then I want you to close the book, take a deep breath, and take that single first step. It is your one and only life. Go live it.

INDEX

food (*continued*)
   and experimenting with herbs and spices,
      430–31
   front-loading with, 415, 434
   gum chewing and, 427–28
   intake of, 166–76
   NEAT activation and, 135–36, 151
   NEAT makeovers and, 117–18, 124–25
   organic, 434–35, 458
   from other countries, 424
   overeating and, 82, 170–71, 175–76
   selection of, 171–74
   shopping for, 439–40
   and steady and predictable fueling, 187–88
   sugary, 172–73, 241, 254, 312, 411–12
   swapping of, 444
   tastes of, 395, 399, 416
   weight and, 79–80, 166–70, 173
   see also NEAT Fuel, NEAT Fueling
friends, 111, 132, 153, 193, 205
   week 1 and, 219, 227, 230, 235
   week 2 and, 259
   week 3 and, 279, 288, 293
   week 4 and, 319
   week 5 and, 370
   week 6 and, 384, 403
   week 7 and, 414, 418, 422
   week 8 and, 438, 447, 451, 460
fruits, 171–81
   citrus, 455

ABOUT THE AUTHOR

James A. Levine, MD, PhD, is a professor of medicine at the Mayo Clinic in Rochester, Minnesota. Professor Levine holds the Richard Emslander Chair in nutrition and in metabolism. He is a professor of physiology and of bioengineering, and he is an internationally renowned expert in obesity.

His research has focused on understanding NEAT, obesity, and body-weight regulation. He has published articles in the most prestigious scientific journals: five articles in *Science* and others in *Nature*, the *New England Journal of Medicine*, and *The Lancet*.

Dr. Levine lectures around the world and is a senior scientific adviser to the U.S. government, the United Nations, and the government of the People's Republic of China as well as throughout Africa and in Jamaica. He is a designated "expert" for the United Nations, NIH, and National Science Foundation. He is an invitee to the

President's Panel.

Based on Dr. Levine's work, articles have appeared in national newspapers and magazines such as *Time*, the *Daily Telegraph*, *U.S. News & World Report*, *Newsweek*, the *New York Times*, the *London Times*, and the *Washington Post* and media in countries as diverse as China, India, Japan, and Poland.

Professor Levine has been interviewed by CNN, NBC, CBS, ABC, BBC, and Fox, and channels in Russia, Australia, and the Far East. He has completed documentaries for the Discovery Channel and BBC. His work has precipitated 2.5 billion-person media hits. He completed his fifth documentary this year.

Professor Levine has received more than fifty national and international awards in science, including the Judson Daland Prize from the American Philosophical Society. He holds multiple NIH grants and federal grants. His walking desk won the invention of the future from NASA and is now a product by Steelcase. His book on NEAT will be published early next year, as will his first novel, entitled *The Blue Notebook*.